Surviving Paris

Surviving Paris

A Memoir of Healing in the City of Light

Robin Allison Davis

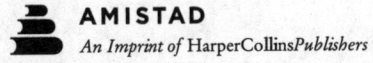

Without limiting the exclusive rights of any author, contributor or the publisher of this publication, any unauthorized use of this publication to train generative artificial intelligence (AI) technologies is expressly prohibited. HarperCollins also exercise their rights under Article 4(3) of the Digital Single Market Directive 2019/790 and expressly reserve this publication from the text and data mining exception.

SURVIVING PARIS. Copyright © 2025 by Robin Allison Davis. All rights reserved. Printed in the United States of America. No part of this book may be used or reproduced in any manner whatsoever without written permission except in the case of brief quotations embodied in critical articles and reviews. For information, address HarperCollins Publishers, 195 Broadway, New York, NY 10007. In Europe, HarperCollins Publishers, Macken House, 39/40 Mayor Street Upper, Dublin 1, D01 C9W8, Ireland.

HarperCollins books may be purchased for educational, business, or sales promotional use. For information, please email the Special Markets Department at SPsales@harpercollins.com.

harpercollins.com

FIRST EDITION

Designed by Kyle O'Brien

Library of Congress Cataloging-in-Publication Data has been applied for.

ISBN 978-0-06-335313-8

25 26 27 28 29 LBC 5 4 3 2 1

For Tiffany Illana Glover:
The world was robbed of your presence, personality,
talent, and humor far too soon. You continue
to be one of my biggest inspirations.

Contents

Disclaimer — ix

1. Best Weekend of My Life — 1
2. *Pourquoi Paris ? Pourquoi Pas Paris !* — 20
3. The Paris Plan — 43
4. Testing, Testing — 59
5. Life Comes at You Fast and So Does Cancer — 70
6. *Playboy* for Breast Cancer and an Amputation — 86
7. You Don't Know What You Don't Know — 103
8. Getting Even: A Tale of Two Titties (They Both Look Good!) — 129
9. Even the Most Beautiful City in the World Can Feel Like the Loneliest — 147

CONTENTS

10. This Is My Year	157
11. The Carousel of Cancer	176
12. Illegitimi Non Carborundum	191
13. The Frozen Five	201
14. And So It Begins	215
15. A Holiday Season Unlike Any Other	235
16. "2 Legit 2 Quit"	246
17. In the Homestretch	252
18. Life Is Short and Long	271
Acknowledgments	285

DISCLAIMER

This is my story, as I remember it.

Surviving Paris

1

Best Weekend of My Life

My feet pounded the cobblestone streets. All around me, families snapped smiling photos and lovers, hand in hand, secured locks on the nearby bridge. Beer bottles tinkled in the distance, the noise mingling with laughter wafting up from the banks of the Seine. The Eiffel Tower illuminated the city, shining its rotating spotlight.

It's no wonder Paris attracts the most tourists out of anywhere in the world: its beauty is enchanting. From the imposing *Cathédrale de Notre Dame* with its snarling gargoyles to the warm glow of the Louvre's glass pyramid, everywhere you turn there's a sight even better than the last.

For two weeks, the city at night was my playground. I would leave my office across the road, drop my work bag inside my front door, change into my beat-up white Chuck Taylors, and hit the streets. I walked for hours, but my feet didn't ache. In fact, I couldn't feel anything at all. Walking, roaming, wandering, often not arriving home until 3 a.m., sleeping only two to three hours before waking to head to work. To start it all over again.

The soles of my Chucks wore down from the many miles of walking with no destination or purpose, as I tried to block out the thoughts in my head by doing the only thing I knew that could relieve some stress.

I roamed from *Rue de la Pompe* in the posh 16th *arrondissement* with its massive Haussmannian stone buildings to the elaborate shop windows of the normally bustling department stores on *Boulevard Haussmann* in the 9th to the street buskers performing at Saint-Michel in the 5th, my eyes drinking in as much as they could.

People flagged down taxis and staggered to catch the last Métro train of the night. I inhaled the sweet smell of batter, as men in aprons cooked crêpes on street corners. It almost made up for the smell of urine, persistent in certain parts of the city, especially this time of night.

I skirted tourists taking photos, not wanting my face, ghostlike and solemn, in the background. I watched stores lock up for the evening, pulling down their heavy metal gates. All for a few hours of distraction from the good night's sleep I knew would never come. I was in a trance—almost sleepwalking—but also intoxicated and overwhelmed by the sights.

The weather was crisp but not cold. Spring had arrived in the city and all I needed was my trench coat, wrapped tightly around me. I tied it tight, then tighter, and even tighter, not only to shield myself from the midnight breeze but also to hold me in its embrace like a security blanket.

As I tied my coat, my arm brushed lightly against my chest. The imposter was still there.

I was waiting on my biopsy results.

"There's no way a doctor would make you wait two weeks if the lump was malignant," my friends said.

Everyone assured me it would be okay—the two weeks of torture would end my nightmare. After being poked and prodded, after multiple medical tests and sleepless nights—on June 25, 2018, for better or for worse, I would know my fate. The nightmare could end, or a new chapter would begin.

Anxiety gripped me every single moment of the day and insomnia gripped me every single night. Arriving back at my small split-level studio at 3 a.m., I climbed the steep, winding stairs to the lofted sleeping area. I lay awake in the darkness, hoping for a tiny bit of rest. Some nights, sleep came fast—albeit a restless sleep plagued with nightmares. Other nights, I stared at the sloped ceiling, a mere two feet from my face, silent tears rolling down my cheeks, hoping that sleep, or the dawn, would soon come.

Open any "American in Paris" book and you'll read how on their second day in the City of Light, at a charming outdoor café, over a latte with a foamy heart in the middle, they locked eyes with a dashing young Parisian man who would sweep them off their feet.

Let me tell you—this ain't that story.

I moved to Paris and all I got was breast cancer.

◆ ◆ ◆

TWO WEEKS. FOURTEEN DAYS. LONGEST wait of my life.

I had noticed the lump in March—a roundish, rippled patch near my nipple. With early morning crust still in the corners of my eyes, my fingers grazed the lump while fumbling around with my bra. Half asleep and yawning, I touched it cautiously, then pressed it with my fingertips. Close enough to be part of my areola, but not exactly.

My body stiffened and my blood ran cold at my discovery—waking me up quicker than coffee. I swallowed hard, heart thudding in my ears, and ripped off my bra, flinging it to the floor. Gazing at the lacy black bra, I recoiled in horror, as if the bra were the one to blame, like her lacy details formed the lump personally. I had never felt anything like that before. Sure, sometimes there was a little painful stinging sensation on that same breast, but never a lump.

Standing in my apartment, I inhaled deeply. I needed to take action and be certain that what I felt was real. At age thirty-three, I never knew how to do a breast self-exam—I was often told I was too young to seriously worry about it, wait until you're forty. But standing in my tiny studio, chest heaving, I launched into a hasty exam, moving my fingers in the circular pitter-patter movements I saw on Breast Cancer Awareness Month ads. My fingers paused at the lump—yes, there was definitely something there.

But was this what a lump was supposed to feel like? My fingers pressed harder into my skin. It wasn't smooth like a pinball or dimpled like a golf ball or orange peel—things

I heard lumps could feel like. It felt like an abnormality, a ridged mass—something that could be cleared up if I reduced my stress or even moisturized my skin better. Maybe it was an areola skin issue, instead of an actual lump—why would it be a lump? I was young, healthy, and no one in my family—on both sides—had ever had breast cancer.

Satisfied with my self-diagnosis, I flung on a dress, rushing to be seated and smiling at my desk by 9 a.m. I didn't have the luxury of letting my imagination run away from me. Every morning as I sleepily dressed for work, my fingers brushed against the lump, but I shuttered it out of my mind.

It was so easy to explain away, so easy to put off. Life was too hectic to spend time pondering this situation.

Now that I finally had obtained a job in Paris, I daydreamed of starting a new relationship, maybe meeting the love of my life in a *boulangerie*, like so many other expat women had. I daydreamed about things as basic as finally achieving perfect, accentless French, mastering the throaty *R* sound. I daydreamed of receiving a second job offer—one in the TV industry, the industry I missed every day.

But every morning, my fingertips grazed the lump. And every morning, I threw my bra on and headed out the door to hit the streets of Paris, pushing the lump back to the far reaches of my mind. That's not to say it didn't worry me at all, but the pain was more concerning. In the middle of the day, in the safety of daylight and my office, waiting until my coworkers were away from my open-area computer screen,

I would slyly google "breast cancer + pain." Over and over, Google reassured me that pain is not a common symptom of breast cancer.[*]

I took my problem to the highest levels of counsel: the all-knowing group chat with my girls, cheekily entitled "Sister Circle."

I fired off a flurry of messages.

"Y'all. I've got this weird thing in my boob—I don't think it's a lump though."

"What does it feel like?" Mariah, always first to reply, asked.

"It doesn't feel smooth, it feels bumpy—but I don't think it's a lump because it's painful. I googled and they say that you don't have pain with breast cancer," I responded.

"You know eating a lot of almonds and nuts can cause lumpy breasts—I've had that," Kasey said. "Are you near your period?"

The period question crossed my mind often—it was an easy explanation. As the sharp, shooting pain coursed through my left breast without warning, I checked my period app to see where I fell in my menstrual cycle. With a seven-day period, out of a four-week month, generally, you're *always* near your period. "Oh, it's coming in a week" or "it just finished" was my typical reply—which was true. Boob pain + period = no problem. After all, I had no family history of breast cancer, so the idea seemed foreign.

---

[*] Pain in the breast is now associated more commonly with breast cancer.

Surviving Paris

❖ ❖ ❖

THE LIFE I HAD IN Paris wasn't what I anticipated when I decided to make the move. It wasn't even the life I'd prepared for. But I knew I had to make sacrifices to pursue the life I wanted—the life I wanted to leave my home country for. Going back to school at age thirty-two for a master's degree in global communications at the American University of Paris was not on my life bingo card—I hated school. Too much homework, too much studying, too many books written by people I couldn't relate to. But my dream life required sacrifices—sacrifices beyond what I expected or was prepared for.

After earning my master's at the American University of Paris, I chased the dream of a full-time job—a full-time job in Paris. I was a television journalist in the US and I loved it. It was my dream job that I'd worked toward my entire life. There was nothing like the thrill of bringing stories to life on network television, for thousands, even millions, to watch. I had even won a News and Documentary Emmy for my work several years earlier.

I wanted to do the same work in Paris, but with an international twist: producing international stories for a different audience. Before moving, everyone told me that it would be easy—I'd be a shoo-in for news organizations looking for journalists who are native English speakers. Expectation versus reality was like a bucket of cold water to the face. I arrived in August 2016 to an abysmal French job market.

I suited up and applied where I could with my limited

French. I took an intense news test at an English-language TV station. When I mentioned my Emmy Award in my interview, they told me they had no idea what that was.

In the end, they offered me a freelance job paying eighty euros a day—before taxes were taken out. "But not every day, and you can't take another job because we need you fully available when we call," they explained. I mumbled my gratitude for the offer and shuffled out of the office in the Parisian suburbs. After a notable ten-year career as a journalist in the US, this was humiliating. And I got the feeling that the humiliation wasn't a cultural misunderstanding—they took pleasure in it.

Not only would the equivalent of seventy-five dollars a day not come close to paying my rent, it also wouldn't make a dent in paying back Uncle Sam for the student loans I took out for my graduate degree. I needed to pivot—and pivot fast. My money was running out and my time to secure a job, a future, in Paris was as well.

I interned, unpaid, in communications at UNESCO for four months to complete my two-year master's program. I hoped it would lead to a job—salvation from the wretched job market. I sat at my desk slack-jawed in the UNESCO headquarters as the US announced they were pulling their membership from the organization. "Do I have to pack up and leave now?" I asked my bosses. Nervous and awkward chuckles abounded at the clear anxiety on my face. "Not now, no . . . but we can't hire you after this internship ends," they explained ruefully.

I applied for other jobs, rarely scoring interviews. My

career experience didn't seem to translate well to the French job market. Not to mention, many of the job postings shockingly stated that they only wanted applicants from specific schools—and mine was not listed. It was humbling—humbling and embarrassing. When I was planning to move to Paris, "inability to find a job" wasn't one of my biggest fears. I was hirable—at least in my eyes.

When the job interviews dried up, I took one last internship at an international political communications agency—this one paid, at least, though not very much—hoping my luck would change.

The hustle was *on*. After all, my time in Paris could be coming to an end. I was possibly in my last few months of living in Paris—a city I sacrificed so much to move to and stay in. A city so many of my classmates had left because of a lack of job opportunities and residency options. I interned for another four months, chasing the dangling carrot of a full-time job. "If you prove yourself and do well, I'm sure we can find a work contract for you," my boss said.

Working as a video intern after my esteemed career wasn't my dream job, but I knew I had to be flexible to stay long term. I spent long nights at the office, producing a high-profile video—one that my boss insisted needed to be spectacular to show how "investing in video is something we need to continue." Work politics, you know.

I extended my seven-hundred-and-fifty-euros-per-month internship for one more month, based on the handshake promise from my boss that if he had a little more time, he'd convert it into a suitable job. If I didn't work hard, push myself to the limits to turn this internship into a job, it would be time for me to leave. Time to buckle down, show off, and do what I do best—get it done.

I worked all the time—weekends, late nights until 1 or 2 a.m.—in an environment unlike any I'd ever known. I was a fish out of water—the workplace was extraordinarily international, with everyone speaking multiple languages fluently while I struggled to improve my French, listening intently in the meetings where the spoken language could switch between English and French from speaker to speaker, sometimes sentence to sentence. One coworker even liked to speak to me in Spanish—a language I minored in at university—just to keep me on my toes. I left the office mentally exhausted every night. The pressure was omnipresent. I was no stranger to pressure from my TV days, but this was different. My livelihood, and my dream, were on the line. I had to secure the job in less than three months or else I would be headed back to the US.

The exhaustion was worth it when the video was a hit and I was rewarded with a four-month work contract, with the promise that "If you do well, we can get you a longer, more official contract."

Praise came from all sides, which was nice, but even as the new Multimedia Executive Producer, my salary was still a sixty percent pay cut from my previous New York City television job. But that's okay—because I did it. It's the life I chose, I reminded myself, crawling into bed at night. I achieved my "international career" dream, even if it could only last for four months. It didn't matter that I was being strung along, thrown crumbs to keep me on the line.

The pressure wasn't entirely released, but it lessened. I still had to "prove myself" to earn stability in France. It would either pay off in the end, or I would go back to the US, tail between my legs but with two years of expat living under my belt.

Was it still low paid? Better than the seven hundred and fifty euros, but yes. Would I gain the respect of my colleagues, going from an intern in her thirties to a coworker? That had yet to be seen. Spoiler alert: not really. But all my stress over the past few months paid off. I could relax and enjoy the start of a new chapter of my life in France—and who knows what that could bring?

I was settling into the job, but I still didn't have work friends. I craved a social connection—when everyone scurried off to lunch with colleagues, I often ate alone at my desk, poking at a sad Carrefour-bought salad. To meet people, I placed a candy dish on my desk, if you could call it that—just a small card table situated in the hallway corner between filing cabinets.

As people walked by or stopped to talk to my colleagues, their eyes inevitably wandered over to my candy dish for an afternoon sugar rush. No one wants to be the rude person grabbing candy from a coworker's desk without a hello or how are you—my candy dish relied on their sweet tooth and manners to force introductions. It was a catalyst for a few awkward conversations but also helped shape a few workplace friendships.

"We're all going out for drinks on Friday night if you want to join. We'll probably go dancing after," said Chelsea, a Canadian coworker I'd become friendly with. She had no idea her invitation made my entire day. "Oh, really?" I said, playing it cool. "Well, I have plans this weekend, but I think I can make it work. I'd love to join."

And it was true—some friends were coming to Paris for *Dîner en Blanc*, the exclusive dress-all-in-white pop-up dinner party. It was the thirtieth anniversary of the invite-only international event—which started in Paris—and was expected to be a once-in-a-lifetime experience.

We planned our attendance for months, poring over past pictures, searching for the right outfit and table. It was also the second weekend of *Roland Garros*, the tennis Grand Slam tournament also known as the French Open. Since my arrival in France two years earlier, I made it a point to go to every year. Every evening I checked my *Roland Garros* app for last-minute tickets to see Serena Williams play—one of her first tournaments back after her difficult childbirth. I scored a pretty good seat for her Saturday third-round match against the German player Julia Görges. It was a bucket list experience for me.

This weekend was going to be epic—which was well-deserved considering how many nights and weekends I had spent holed up staring at Adobe Premiere.

That Friday, I put special care into choosing an outfit. I wanted to become part of this friend circle, so if I needed to be the last person standing on the dance floor, I would do it. And honestly, it doesn't take much for me to be the last person standing on the dance floor. Or the first person, either, for what it's worth. I had been known to get the party started at a wedding or two.

We hopped from bar to bar, crisscrossing Paris by Métro, singing along to music at the top of our lungs. We danced, we laughed, we sang, we talked, we drank, and I was deliriously happy. I missed having a work community—in NYC my office often frequented the Rockefeller Center Rink Bar after finishing grueling assignments—and this had the same feel.

We kept the party going as we returned to Chelsea's Montmartre apartment, discussing everything from work to the meaning of life to my coworker's particularly luscious man bun and hair routine. I caught the first train of the day, yawning at 5 a.m. on the platform. I was exhausted and bleary eyed but happy. Today was a good day.

On Saturday, the sun's intensity didn't stop me from crossing off my bucket list item. I arrived at *Roland Garros*, sundress on and straw hat in hand to beat the heat of the day. Entering the Suzanne Lenglen court a few minutes before the match, I walked down the steep stairs to my seat—which, to my surprise, was only nine rows from the iconic red-clay court. Used to American ticket prices, I had no idea that a hundred and ninety euros bought fantastic seats. The same ticket price at the US Open would have me zooming into the court on my phone's camera.

The ninety-degree heat couldn't stop goosebumps from prickling my arms when Serena walked out on the court in her black catsuit with a wide red midriff. I pinched myself. I could smell the court; I could see the furrow of Serena's brow during a difficult serve. I could hear every grunt, every frustrated exhalation. It was thrilling. She won the match, a big win for her after her health challenges. I looked at her with childlike wonder, inspired by her athleticism, her spirit, after all she went through. I bounded down the stairs after the match and asked a stranger to snap a photo of me by the court. My face hurt from smiling so hard. I would remember this day forever. Today was a good day.

By the time Sunday rolled around, I woke up with a smile on my face. I had heard so many good things about *Dîner en Blanc*—and it was good timing that my friend Tommy was in town. *Dîner en Blanc* was not your normal dinner party; it required work—the only dinner party in the world where you not only have to dress in all white but also have to not get your all-white outfit dirty while lugging your food, drinks, table, chairs, and cutlery to the secret location announced only an hour prior. I was grateful to have Tommy with me as a bit of muscle.

Getting dressed in my awkwardly laid-out apartment in the 16th arrondissement, I caught my eye in the mirror and smiled at myself. Despite everything I was up against, I had actually done it. I had gone back to school at thirty-two, in a foreign country whose language I didn't know. I earned my master's degree, completing far too many irksome group projects and reading numerous theoretical communications books, about which my professors insisted, "You'll need this someday; you'll use this in your future jobs."

I had invested in my future, taking the unpaid internship and then a low-paid internship, even switching apartments to lower my expenses. I did all of these things with the goal of having an international career, and I achieved it. I landed a job in Paris. I finally turned a corner, and I was so ready for all the good that would come my way.

I slipped into a white V-neck jumpsuit, one I found in the back of my closet, but perfect for the event.

Carrying salads, cutlery, tables, and chairs, we departed for *Dîner en Blanc*. This year's secret location was *Esplanade des Invalides*, the lawn in front of the gilded military complex that houses Napoleon's tomb. Throngs of people dressed in white traipsed across the grass, toting everything from dining chairs to candelabras and elaborate centerpieces. We danced until our feet ached, sinking into the soft dirt of the esplanade. The night ended with champagne and sparklers, revelry in full swing. I couldn't keep a smile off of my face. My cup was incredibly full. I was content. Today was a good day.

I walked into work Monday morning, still riding a high. "Good morning, Robin. How was your weekend?" my coworker asked. "It was the best weekend of my life," I responded, plopping down at my desk with a smile. Her eyebrows lifted in surprise. "Wow, sounds like a good weekend," she said, and laughed. And it really was.

I was finally going up on the elevator of life, after pressing the up button repeatedly, without progress. I was on the rise in all aspects after feeling stagnant for so long: I was starting my career; I was making new friends. Who knows—maybe I could even find love next?

My life in Paris was good, even with the bumps in the road. The elevator was on the move again. The lump was the furthest thing from my mind.

That afternoon, I planned to leave work early for my annual pap smear. I'd seen my gynecologist a few months prior, so it would be a quick in-and-out appointment.

◆ ◆ ◆

WITH MY WORK CONTRACT IN hand, three months after feeling the lump, I could try to figure things out. I always took good care of my health when insured—so now that I had a bit of breathing room, I could start my regular checkups. I booked a checkup appointment with my gynecologist.

Doctor's appointments in France were always an "experience" and gynecological visits were no different. Doctors' offices were often in apartment buildings—sometimes tucked away on the side on the ground floor but often right smack-dab in the middle on a floor of personal apartments. Checking in with the receptionist? There often isn't one: you walk into a waiting room after being buzzed in, hoping that the doctor is running on time and will retrieve you when they're free.

Some doctors claimed to be bilingual, able to receive English-speaking patients. It was definitely an exaggeration when, two months after arriving in France, I visited a dermatologist who, after examining me, sat me down and told me with great concern in halting English, "You have mushrooms." I panicked until we came to the understanding that he meant a skin fungus.

Other doctors refused to join the twenty-first century, which I discovered during my first physical appointment in France. I regretted my choice of doctor the minute I stepped into the cramped office with towering open boxes of paperwork—patient files—scattered all over the floor. She spent several minutes rustling through her boxes of papers to find a clean intake form for me. Good luck ever asking to see your file.

If you had to disrobe at a doctor's office, the comfort of privacy was also nonexistent. At my first gynecological appointment in France, the male doctor pointed me to a corner of his office to undress. Space is at a premium in Paris, and the exam table and doctor's desk are often in the same room, separated by a screen, sometimes only mere feet away from each other. Thank God that eating lunch at your desk is frowned upon in France. And unlike in the US, a female nurse isn't present for your comfort and safety. Just the septuagenarian French doctor and me with my pants off (gowns or coverings were never provided), being told to spread 'em wide. Suffice to say, I was never particularly eager to go to the doctor in France.

But this doctor was different, thankfully. Dr. Boucher came referred—she was a favorite of many Americans in Paris. She had the comforts of home, like a receptionist and a private area to disrobe in. Meticulous and direct, her dry, flat affect also reminded me of home—more specifically of so many of the women I knew in NYC. You could tell that she doesn't scare easily. And the best part? She was perfectly bilingual. This doctor, I liked.

After work, I hopped on the Métro toward her office in the 7th arrondissement, not far from the Eiffel Tower and the university where I did my studies.

The lump was still the furthest thing from my mind. Still riding a high from my weekend, I didn't think this doctor's appointment would interrupt my recent spate of good fortune. I hoisted myself up on the leather exam table, not offering any information about what I felt or had been experiencing. A small part of me suppressed my worries and wanted to delay the moment—the moment when she would do my breast exam and possibly change the course of my life. Anxiety didn't course through my veins; I wasn't waiting with bated breath. Everything would be fine—it had to be. I'd had a few hiccups in my life, but for the most part, it had always turned out well.

"Okay, sit up and move to the edge of the table," Dr. Boucher instructed in her lightly accented English. I raised my arms and she ran her fingers over my right breast, then my left. Her brow furrowed as her fingers pressed into my left breast. I watched intently, noticing that she was taking longer on the left than the right. She repeated the exam on the left breast, then leaned back and exhaled.

"There's something here; have you felt this before?"

My face flushed with shame, my cheeks reddening as much as a Black woman's could.

"I felt something there, but I wasn't sure what it was," I

admitted. It sounded so much worse saying it aloud. I was embarrassed.

"Let's get a few tests done, so we can see what it is," she said, leaving the exam area and walking to her desk. I searched her face with my eyes, looking for a hint, any indication of what she thought. But my gynecologist, who I liked for her directness and lack of emotion, gave no signs of what was to come.

I sat back in my chair as she wrote out prescription after prescription. Suddenly, my week filled up with appointment after appointment. "First, you go get an MRI and a mammogram," she explained. "Then we'll do a sonogram and biopsy." I nodded dumbly, taking the papers into my hand. "After that, you come back here for an appointment and we'll discuss."

Discuss, I thought, turning it over in my mind. There should be nothing to discuss. Nothing at all. But as it turns out, I was beginning my whirlwind adventure through the French medical system.

2

Pourquoi Paris ? Pourquoi Pas Paris !

"I hated Paris. It's not the place for me," I haughtily proclaimed to friends, family, anyone who would listen.

March 1997—I was a quiet, skinny, chocolate-brown girl with a Just for Me relaxer done in her grandma's Washington, DC, kitchen, an awkward gait, glasses as big as her face, and honestly, a nose to match. I wasn't tall but somehow still gangly—all legs. My teeth were a disaster, with canines that hung down like a vampire's and two side teeth that had decided to do their own thing. If we're keeping it real, I had a face only a mother could love.

But this little girl was a dreamer. Nestled away under her love of reading, writing, and theater hid a quiet sense of adventure. A sense of adventure that was stoked by a school trip at the age of twelve.

I attended a small religious school—my sixth-grade class was only thirteen students and most of us had known each other since kindergarten. Our school didn't have a ton of resources. We didn't have every sports team known to man, a flashy cafeteria, or multiple foreign-language classes to choose from. We didn't have famous alumni or art facilities. But we did have teachers who cared, a lot. My Spanish teacher, Mrs. Gibbs, decided she would take as many of us sheltered Maryland students as she could on a ten-day European trip over spring break—to London, Paris, and Madrid.

Europe had never crossed my mind as a place where I could actually step foot one day—it seemed like a faraway place I couldn't relate to. A place you read about in history books, learning about old white men who were long dead, but not a place with living history.

My friends and I gossiped in the back of the church sanctuary—it doubled as our school auditorium—as our parents attentively listened to Mrs. Gibbs's extensive presentation. I pitched forward slightly in my chair, as she explained how after London, we'd take the ferry across the English Channel and then a bus to head into Paris.

My curiosity piqued, I started listening, blocking out my friends' tittering. The Eiffel Tower and Seine River appeared on the screen, faded photos flickering from the projector, but it didn't matter—I was sold. I had to make this trip. Plus, it was geared toward the high schoolers, and my friends and I desperately wanted to go—if not to see Europe, then to spend a few days mooning over our crushes outside of the confines of school.

At twelve, I wasn't a world traveler. I had flown only twice before in my life: a trip to Disney World when I was eight and a family cruise from Mexico. My travel experience was mostly limited to road trips to South Carolina to go to family funerals. My parents would tack on extra days for the drive back to swing by Myrtle Beach for some beach and miniature golf time. If I was lucky, they'd acquiesce to my pleas to stop by South of the Border, the tacky Mexican-themed strip mall in South Carolina, on the way back up to Maryland.

This trip would be completely different, and I had to go. I pleaded with my parents to swing the high cost of the trip. "Please? I really want to go. We'll have chaperones! The deposit is due soon," I begged like a broken record. "We'll see," was my parents' response—a response that irked me, since it was so common in our household. As we inched toward the deposit date, my pleading ramped up until one evening, my parents sat me down at the dining room table for a discussion.

My father started, always speaking measured and slow.

"We know that you're interested in this Europe trip with the school," he began.

"Yes, yes," I said, urging him to pick up the pace. The suspense was killing me.

"Now, your mother and I decided," he said, locking eyes with my mother and gesturing toward her, "that you can go, but only if Mom comes with you as a chaperone."

I exhaled and my face lit up in excitement. "Thank you thank you thank you!"

Not the best scenario I had in mind as a preteen who did everything in her power to avoid being near her parents, but definitely a winning scenario overall. I ran to the kitchen, yanking the yellow phone off the receiver, eager to tell my friends my good news. They all had good news too—since my mom was going, their parents felt comfortable sending them on the trip as well.

Landing in London, I felt like I was in a different world. The posh accents made me giggle or sometimes stare in confusion—they *are* speaking English, right? The buildings were older than anything I'd seen in the US. I couldn't wrap my head around how ancient it all looked to my twelve-year-old self. Double-decker buses zoomed down the opposite side of the road, both frightening and thrilling me. Everything seemed louder, busier, and more vibrant than in DC.

Even the music was different—in every store we entered, from every radio we passed by, we heard the same raspy voice crooning "Don't speak, I know what you're thinking," from a song that we'd never heard before but was obviously a chart-topper in England. By the end of our days in London, we'd all know the words to it. Years later, I'd become a big fan of the group No Doubt, their song "Don't Speak" transporting me back fondly to my first time abroad. The dreary skies and constant drizzle of rain did nothing to quell my excitement. I was in Europe, a place I never expected I'd see.

As we traversed the London streets, a group of twenty Black students aged eleven to seventeen, there was a familiar refrain.

"Oh, what a lovely group! You're a choir?"

"What a group of well-behaved students—where is your basketball tournament?"

Each time we gently explained to Londoners that no, we were not a choir or a basketball team. It was unfathomable to people that we, a group of Black American students, would be on an educational trip of this scale. We zipped around the city on a grueling tour schedule, led by Andy, our fearless British guide. By the end of the trip, I bought a souvenir stuffed animal and nicknamed him Andy—he had become like part of the family after so many days and nights together. Our days were packed with multiple museum visits, and by the end of each night we fell asleep easily, much to the relief of our chaperones.

Following a whirlwind London visit, we arrived in Paris after a long bus and ferry ride across the English Channel past the white cliffs of Dover. There was an immediate change in the air: the skies were slightly less dreary but the drizzle was persistent. But it wasn't just the weather—the vibe was different from London. People weren't rushing to their workplaces; they were having leisurely lunches at the cafés. They were enjoying a glass of wine at midday, slim cigarette in hand, people-watching at the street-facing tables. The French gave off an air of being effortlessly cool, not fussed, and would never deign to rush about town like the Londoners we had just experienced.

The Haussmannian buildings—in the iconic French architecture style of grand stone structures popular for their angled slate-gray metal rooftops, colorful oversized doors, and iron balconies—were impressive. Unlike London, the city didn't have skyscrapers; in fact, it reminded us of DC—a city designed by Frenchman Pierre Charles L'Enfant—with its low buildings, all eight floors or less.

Gazing upon the Iron Lady herself—the Eiffel Tower—was a trip highlight. We took the elevator up to the top and walked the sixteen hundred plus iron stairs back down to the bottom. My mother snapped a picture of me in front of the Eiffel Tower—I was wearing an ill-fitting leather jacket, hers from her teenage years. Huge glasses sat crookedly on my face, and I wore an even bigger smile. We walked the bridges traversing the Seine River—there were so many of them—some with wooden planks and others with golden fixings. We explored Paris, hopping from neighborhood to neighborhood, known as *arrondissements*. They were laid out in a spiral shape, like escargot, numbering from the 1st arrondissement with the Louvre wrapping around to the 20th arrondissement with the Père Lachaise Cemetery. It was different from anything I'd ever known.

Different, but not necessarily better.

The amazement and wonder I felt upon landing in London wasn't present in Paris. What was present was dog poop, and lots of it. We walked on the streets of Paris like a live-action version of Frogger, sidestepping, dodging, and watching the ground for the brown, steaming piles. We saw more evidence of dogs than the actual dogs themselves.

Nothing could have prepared me for my trip to Paris—it was a comedy of errors. Every day, we piled into a bus for sightseeing, stopping to have lunch at various Parisian restaurants. One day, lunch started with a bang—quite literally. I entered the busy café and was led past the dining Parisians to our section in the back by the waitstaff. The café was full—the lunch crowd had already arrived—and I was eager to sit down for a meal after a long morning of museums. Eager—perhaps too eager.

We arrived at our table, complete with a white tablecloth. As I bent to take my seat, the waiter pulled out my chair simultaneously with a flourish. *"Mademoiselle."* I crashed to the floor of the busy restaurant, landing loudly for everyone to hear. My gangly limbs entangled in the chair and table, and my legs scissored in the air in an attempt to free them. I flailed about, the ends of the white tablecloth flying as I tried to stabilize. The entire restaurant paused, forks midair, heads whipping around to catch a glimpse of the ruckus. I scrambled to my feet, brushing off the waiter's cries of *"Mademoiselle, mademoiselle!"* Classy. My cheeks flushed with embarrassment, I was silent for most of the meal, hoping everyone would forget.

Strike one, Paris.

The following day, I hoped my shame was behind me. At twelve years old, few things are more embarrassing than a graceless fall—especially in front of upperclassmen, who did not attempt to hide their laughter. I was mortified, trying to fade into the background until the whole thing was forgotten.

Thankfully, we focused on the day's touristic activities instead of all the social points I'd lost the day before. We boarded *Le Bateau-Mouche* for a sightseeing boat ride down the Seine River. Notre Dame and the *Musée D'Orsay* floated past us, and we snapped pictures with our disposable and film cameras. We waved at Parisians enjoying picnics on the banks of the river; some kind enough to wave back at us.

Our chaperones stayed to themselves, enjoying adult conversation and not having to worry about us running off somewhere during the hour-long cruise. Screams erupted from our group—high-pitched shrieks turned to laughter—when halfway through the ride we were mooned from the banks of the Seine. After we had waved at a group of male Parisians from the boat, they had turned around and dropped their pants to give us a unique view of the French, bare pasty bums wiggling at us with abandon. We screamed and laughed in delight, some of us snapping photos, as our chaperones ran to cover our eyes and turn our heads.

Strike two, Paris (or was it really?).

The whole trip wasn't just bus and boat rides. Andy corralled us onto the Métro, for the real Parisian experience. The Parisian subway system, much like the DC Metro that we were used to, was efficient and relatively safe. We crowded into the station, following the universal rules of commuting: walk to the right, stand to the left, and wait at the sides of the door for passengers to exit first. The green and white train barreled into the station, noisy and packed with commuters. I stepped to the side, waiting patiently for others to exit, when a man flew out of the car, turned to the side, and punched me full force in the stomach. I flew backward into the crowd, clutching my stomach and gasping for air. The man, wild-eyed and manic, pivoted to kick my friend in the leg and ran out of the station, ignoring the shouts in both French and English. Bewildered and in pain, I nodded weakly to all the concerned Parisians crowding around me asking if I was okay.

So let me get this straight. An embarrassing fall, a mooning, and then an assault?

Paris, strike three, you're out.

I exhaled in relief when we finally boarded the train at *Gare Montparnasse* to continue to our next leg of the trip—Madrid. My Paris experience had stressed me out, and I looked forward to our long ride to Spain. But as I bought my sandwich for the ten-hour-plus train ride, Paris had one last surprise for me. As the train rocked back and forth, an American passenger walked through the car, speaking with my teachers to kill time. Just as I unwrapped my baguette sandwich, the train rocked violently, tossing the woman onto my lap and on top of my unwrapped sandwich. She flailed (much as I had done in the restaurant, ironically) on top of all ninety-nine pounds of me—well, me plus my sandwich. When she finally regained her footing, she apologized profusely, gazing down at the sandwich that now resembled a quesadilla.

After that trip, I knew I had had enough of Paris for a lifetime. It's hard to imagine that the awkward preteen who proclaimed that she hated Paris would grow up to move there as an adult to start a new chapter in her life. Perhaps this trip was the first indication that I would love a city that, at times, didn't feel like it loved me back.

♦ ♦ ♦

AFTER MY FIRST TRIP TO Paris, over twenty years ago, it's easy to see that moving to Paris was never my dream. I'm not the woman who watched *Amélie* on repeat with stars in her eyes—in all honesty, I couldn't even get through one viewing of it. I'm not the woman who studied French in school—it wasn't even offered until I went to college. I'm not the woman who made Julia Child recipes or adored French food—I preferred to eat Mexican, Thai, and Chinese instead. But moving to Paris wasn't just a whim either.

Every morning I woke up in my NYC apartment feeling less and less fulfilled. At thirty-one years old, I had a great career doing what I loved, but in the back of my brain, there was a nagging feeling that I needed more. Wanted more. For ten years I traveled the world, booking and conducting interviews, field producing, and pulling together numerous hours of television documentaries. I did everything from interviewing A-list celebs like Angelina Jolie to hidden-camera bar shoots to climbing twelve-foot vertical ladders to sail on a cargo freighter.

Was it exciting? Sure, but I wanted more. I aspired to produce on an international level—giving a voice to the voiceless worldwide. I'd worked on an award-winning piece on child soldiers in the Democratic Republic of Congo, but those stories were few and far between. I didn't think I was the second coming of Christiane Amanpour or Soledad O'Brien, but I wanted to do more. I was too comfortable—from my bright and cozy Harlem apartment that I lived in for eight years to my job that I could have done blindfolded with one arm tied behind my back.

Weekends were fun, but routine. Saturday mornings in Harlem, I'd meet up with friends for boozy mimosa brunches, catching up on life, frequently cackling in laughter at everything from dating to wacky coworker stories. At night, we frequented the same lounges and restaurants, even making friends with the bouncers and bartenders.

The weekend would end with a stroll in Central Park, just ten animated city blocks from my apartment. I considered it my backyard. It was one of my favorite places in NYC and a reason I loved living in Harlem. I walked the tree-lined concrete path in the park, often pausing to sit near the water at the Harlem Meer, to settle my mind and get fresh air before the "Sunday scaries" started.

Every couple of months, I rode Amtrak down to DC to see my family, and I was even starting to see the same guys over and over on the dating apps, sometimes swiping right to say a little hello and chuckle at our rematch, despite having already experienced a first date short on chemistry. My life in Harlem was good. Good but routine.

But the idea of life abroad excited me. I was always drawn to expat stories—reading bloggers recounting their early days in a new country and befriending the expats I met on my travels. I liked the idea of trying something new before settling into the expected wife/mom life—despite the fact that there was no husband or even boyfriend on the horizon.

Above all, I wanted that international career: producing

pieces that impacted more than just the lives of Americans but also the lives of people worldwide. It was a part of my career that was lacking, no matter how many international stories I pitched without success. I was already applying for jobs abroad, but the process always ended abruptly when they asked the dreaded question, "Do you already have a work visa?" Once I answered no, I became an untouchable. No one wanted to sponsor a visa for me to move abroad, so I was never a viable candidate. I faced rejection after rejection.

So was moving abroad really possible? Once I got there, would I be able to find a job? What about dating: was I ruining my chances of finding true love? Not to mention, would racism take a bigger role in my everyday life than it currently did? Moving abroad seemed like something that was for *them*, but not for *us*.

What could life be like if I just changed locales?

Walking through Central Park on a Sunday afternoon, I turned the idea over in my mind. If I could do it, where would I go? What city would be good for me? Earlier in the month, I had gone to London and Switzerland for a shoot. In a diner in Geneva, over greasy overpriced pizza, the topic of moving abroad came up among the London-based camera crew. Nancy, a Canadian producer who had moved to Europe over twenty years ago, listened to me speaking with stars in my eyes about expat life.

"Well, it sounds like you really want to live abroad," she said.

"Definitely. I mean I do, but I don't get how it all works—will I get a job, how will I find a place to live—all of those things. I've been applying for jobs abroad for years but they won't take me because I don't already have a visa," I lamented.

"Just do it. I know so many women who have just done it—you won't regret it. And if it doesn't work out, you just move back. But I'm sure you can figure things out," she encouraged.

Her advice shocked me. I never thought it could be as simple as taking the leap—legally, of course. But now, walking in Central Park on a brisk spring day, the conversation played out again in my head. My mind snapped back to the question "Where would I go?"

To me, New York City is one of the best cities in the world. It had its problems—all cities do—but I loved the city despite the hard times. Why reduce my quality of life by leaving for a tiny town, just for the sake of adventure?

I walked back uptown, still weighing the pros and cons of the situation. I could think of nothing else. On my morning commute to Rockefeller Center, the number 2 train rocking noisily, cramped with straphangers, I tapped out a list in my iPhone of the criteria I wanted for my new city. I knew I wanted a place with lots of diversity, plenty of green spaces (I needed a "Central Park" wherever I lived), free or cheap things to do (in case I was low on funds or unemployed for a bit), and a location not too far from the East Coast, with major airports. I needed good public transport—despite how much the subway annoyed me, I didn't want to buy a car. On the career side, I needed to be in a major city if I wanted to work in international news.

And surprise—writing my list put Paris at the top. I never gave Paris much thought after my childhood experience, despite having visited again as an adult. London was another possibility, but I'd recently soured on the city. I wasn't a fan of the weather, the cost of living, or the food. So I dove into researching Paris—now that I'd settled on a locale, it was time to see how to make this possibility a reality.

I pored over website after website and blog after blog to find out how so many women were making the leap and doing it legally. The majority of the American expat women moved for love—they met a Frenchman abroad, on vacation, on the internet—and moved to Paris to start a life with him. Despite my years of swiping on dating apps, I didn't have any prospects to make this an option for me.

I also had no desire to take an extended vacation and travel out of Europe every three months to reset a tourist visa. I wanted to be fully immersed, have an apartment, my own life—essentially, I wanted my current life, but abroad. After hours of research, I discovered the most common hack for single people looking to move to France seemed to be the easily obtainable student visa.

Many people move to France to learn French—which makes sense—but it was also a route that allowed you to obtain a student visa for a minimum of a year. Despite my desperation to live abroad, though, I didn't want to put my life on hold by taking French lessons.

Driven by my career goals of not only living but also working abroad, I researched master's degree programs in Paris and landed on the website of the American University of Paris's Masters of Global Communications program. The eighteen-month program, entirely in English, boasted of landing jobs around the world for their students. And the best part? It was accredited in Delaware, meaning that I could take out federal student loans to finance my graduate degree. I scrolled the site, looking at the students' smiling faces. Maybe I could be one of them.

It'd been so long since I was in school—and I didn't enjoy it when I was. My time at Howard University was amazing, but it had more to do with the social and community aspects than with the academics. I considered myself a "doer" and less of a classroom learner. Could I really, in my early thirties, almost ten years out of undergrad, go back to school and do it in a foreign country?

Honestly, the answer was *probably*. I never doubted myself when it came to perseverance. I'd worked several internships, all unpaid, to get me to the point of working for NBC News, in a job that I loved. For two years I worked an assistant job at NBC that so closely resembled *The Devil Wears Prada* that I can't watch the movie to this day (it's not a comedy to me!). The six- to seven-day workweeks of seventy hours, coming home to a moldy, roach-infested Harlem apartment that gave me months-long sinus infections that I didn't have real health insurance to get treatment for, had led me to where I was at that very moment: in my light-filled (non-mold- and roach-infested) Harlem apartment, working as a producer, traveling the country for work, and doing a job that I loved and was passionate about.

I lived by the saying: "I can do anything for two years."

If the master's program turned out to be an utter waste of time, at least I would have lived in Paris for two years and finally accomplished a *portion* of the dream. A portion of the dream to the tune of over sixty thousand dollars in student loans. If moving to Paris to start a new life was the hardest thing I'd have to do in my life, then all said, I would have had a great life.

The idea excited me, but I wasn't entirely sold on The Paris Plan. The student loans would be a major undertaking. I wanted to be sure. Perhaps things would work out in the US—maybe I'd finally get that promotion I'd been working toward. After all, I'd rather travel abroad producing international news for work than have to do it on my own dime. I didn't want to be impulsive. I made a list of graduate programs in Paris and set it to the side.

• • •

I LOVED BEING ON THE road. My job required that I travel often and sometimes with not much advance notice. I traveled for shoots, interviews, booking trips, and even murder trials. I lived out of my suitcase for up to a month at a time in places like Kelowna, in British Columbia; Paducah, Kentucky; and Los Angeles. I was chased by a rifle-toting pickup truck driver in Pennsylvania, rolled into a ditch in a freak snowstorm in Kentucky, and pursued a freighter ship in Miami from a skivvy to get the perfect shot (and it was perfect—it was used several times throughout the episode and in the promos). I managed hundreds of hours of footage on-site at the White House, the highlight of my day being able to say hello to Bo Obama, the friendly Portuguese water dog. Wherever the story was, I was ready to go there and hit the ground running.

Due to my eagerness to travel and the ease with which I handled the frantic and sometimes hairy situations on the road, I went on assignment often. But it wasn't enough. If I was doing all of this on top of writing, booking and conducting interviews, and sometimes filming and editing—when would I get a promotion to the title I *really* wanted: field producer?

Year after year at my performance reviews, I received stellar feedback. Each time I would ask, "So what about a field producer title?" "Well, you know we got rid of that position, but if we ever brought it back, you'd be it," my manager responded. Either way, the raises kept coming and I was happy with the majority of the assignments I received.

I shoved The Paris Plan to the back of my mind and decided to focus, in earnest, on growing my career, as much as I could, where I was. People told me how lucky I was to work at a network, and how it must be such a dream. In many ways, it was. But I felt suffocated—stifled. When I lay in bed at night, I wondered if I wasn't allowed to dream bigger. I'm a hard worker and a good journalist, but is this where my career was going to begin—and end?

We were sliding toward summer, the relaxed time at work due to the network schedule and viewership drops. People would rather be out enjoying the sun than parked in front of their televisions watching the news—and I don't blame them. It was a warm May day and the subway hadn't yet reached its full mugginess potential. Commuting to work wasn't the hassle that it would be in August. I walked into 30 Rock, ready to start a slow day at work: a little research, cleanup from a recently aired episode, and diving into potential story pitches.

"Robin—did you hear?" Nikki, my partner in crime and work confidant, leaned over the wall separating our cubicles.

"Hear what? I just got in," I said, my eyes darting around, settling in at my desk.

"They promoted Eric, Mike, and Matthew. They promoted them all to *field producer*."

My hands hovered over my keyboard as my eyes widened in disbelief. Field producer? The title that I was told didn't exist and, if it did, would be mine? I was confused—it didn't make sense to me. Sure, Eric, Mike, and Matthew had become the "stars" of the team—a group of guys that were always sent out first to the biggest and best stories. They did great work—there was no denying that. But why bring the title back now? And why wasn't I considered?

Nikki knew how badly I wanted that role—she listened to my gripes on our daily morning (and sometimes afternoon) coffee breaks. I'd been talking about it for years, constantly requesting feedback from my superiors to improve my work and move up the ladder. I wanted answers—no, I *needed* answers, as to why I wasn't considered. I decided to skip straight to the top—not my manager, but Rachel Park, the executive producer. I started my career as her assistant, and I felt we still had a good rapport. If I couldn't get answers from her, then who else could I talk to?

I scheduled a meeting with her a few days later. I spent the days in the lead-up to the meeting mentally reviewing the bullet points I wanted to cover: how long I'd been working toward that position, how many of my manager reviews mentioned I'd be excellent in that job, and how I was an incredibly reliable and competent producer.

My goal wasn't to change her mind, for her to tell me, "Oh, I completely forgot about you, Robin—here, here's your promotion too," but to gain some sort of timeline, no matter how tentative, for my career advancement. The squeaky wheel gets the oil, and I was determined to turn my squeak into a holler.

On the day of the meeting, I put on a dress I felt confident in. If my nerves failed me, at least I'd look cute in my failure. Wiping my sweaty palms on my dress, I approached her corner office overlooking 6th Avenue. I lightly rapped on her office door.

Rachel wasn't a mean boss at all, but she could be intimidating. You always wanted to be on top of your game when talking to her and not wilting under her fierce gaze. She was smart, quick, and had worked her way up through the ranks fairly in a male-dominated field. And she did it all at a relatively young age and while raising children. She was someone I admired and whose approval mattered to me. It was an odd relationship at times—after all, I'd started as a timid twenty-two-year-old fresh out of college. I answered her calls with a chirpy "Rachel Park's office" for nearly two years. I grabbed her coffee and organized her paperwork. I started my career with her—she'd seen me grow up.

"Hey, Robin, come on in," she said, beckoning me with a wave and a smile.

"Hi, Rachel, thanks so much for having this meeting with me," I started. "I wanted to talk to you about my career trajectory here."

"Understandable, you've been here a while and we're glad to have you. What's on your mind?" she asked.

Here we go. "Well, you know for years I've always been sent out on big stories, working in the field on network specials, breaking news, et cetera. I enjoy that—I love that! And I've always wanted to be a field producer. I mention it in all my reviews, and Elliott [my manager] always says that I'm essentially in that role. And that I'm great in that role. But that the field producer title/position doesn't exist anymore at the show."

I drew in a deep breath. "So, I wondered why when the position was created again, Eric, Mike, and Matthew got that job and I wasn't considered." Boom, there it was. I said the big part out loud. My hands were folded tightly in my lap, nervous energy spasming through my fidgety fingers. It took everything in me not to tap my foot.

Rachel leaned back in her chair. Her eyebrows lifted as I spoke, her face a mix of curiosity and surprise. I couldn't read her. Perhaps it was a point of discussion in the promotion process—or maybe they never thought about me at all. "Yes,

I can understand how you would wonder about that. We did decide to bring back that position, and it's because of all the filming that they do in the field," she said.

Nervousness quickly morphed into frustration. "When I spoke to management about my career in the past, I was told that I needed to learn how to edit video. So I learned it. I do it. Then I was told that to advance, I'd need to learn how to film. So I learned that—I shoot in the field often. So I don't see what the difference is?"

Rachel nodded and then smiled gently at me. "Yes, but they shoot *cinematically*, so that's the difference."

The realization hit me like a ton of bricks. No matter what I did, no matter how hard I tried, the goalposts would continuously move. There's no way I would ever cross the finish line to advance my career. I looked down at my sweaty palms, feeling foolish. Feeling foolish and naïve.

"Okay. I understand," I conceded. It wasn't that I understood the reasoning, it was that I understood that it wouldn't happen for me.

"You know," Rachel said, leaning forward with a slight smile on her face. "Sometimes you have to leave to get what you want."

I stared back at her, my heart racing, trying to make sense of both her smile and advice. Swallowing hard, I thanked her for her time and exited her office. I grabbed my purse and walked out of the doors of Rockefeller Center. It was only 4:30, but who cares? When your boss, the one who has the power to advance your career, advises you to find another job, does leaving at 4:30 matter? I was crushed. I'd put too much faith in the idea that if I kept my head down and did what they wanted of me, I'd get to where I wanted to be. And it had worked, for a while. It got me to where I was. But it was obvious that it wasn't going to get me to where I wanted to be.

Blinking back tears, I pushed my way onto the uptown D train, heading directly to Maison Harlem. Located on a bustling corner of the famed 125th Street, the low-key French restaurant and bar was just the place I needed. I entered the restaurant and the chaos of Harlem on a late spring day faded away. The black and white Parisian bistro's charm enveloped me. The barman smiled warmly and welcomed me in, a reminder that I was, in fact, not in Paris, but in the US.

Sidling up to the bar, I ordered my first French 75—gin, champagne, lemon juice, and simple syrup. It would be the drink of choice that night. I lost myself in thought, swirling the cocktail around in the flute. If my own boss wouldn't see a future for me—couldn't see a future for me—then how could I? "Another, please," I said, flagging down the bartender.

And I sat. I sat there in my shame, in my embarrassment, in my naïveté, drinking French 75 after French 75. My friend Cassandra joined me after a couple of rounds, alternately offering supportive words and sitting in sympathetic silence. She left to go home after a few drinks, leaving me in my funk. I sat at the bar at the beginning of happy hour, the early crowd strolling in to meet friends. I sat at the bar from the end of happy hour to dinnertime, watching couples and families seated for a French dining experience. I sat at the bar, tears rolling down my face. The bartender slid me a glass of champagne, his face a mix of commiseration and pity.

The meeting was a gut punch—but was it worth being a sniveling, drunken mess? Maybe not. In fact, certainly not. But I felt like a failure. And as I sat there alone in my thoughts, my body was racked with grief. Grieving the idea that I'd continue to move onward and upward at the job I loved. Grieving the idea that if you do everything right—work hard, keep your head down and nose clean—everything works out in the end. Grieving the idea that my life in NYC could change and be more than what I currently had. It was so obvious that my face was pressed against a glass ceiling—and unless I made a major change, I would be stuck. Stuck and bitter, something I'd seen before and had no desire to be.

I left the bar, stumbling the seven blocks back to my apartment. The decision was clear. It was clear the minute I boarded the D train to Harlem. It was clear the minute I stepped into Maison Harlem and the bartender greeted me with *"Bonjour."* My tears weren't just grief but also fear. Fear that I knew what my next step should be: a big, risky next step that could turn out to be a mistake. But the only way to find out is to do it. Life was too short to sit around and hope things would change. If I wanted my life to be different, I would have to take risks.

And I would do it. The Paris Plan would go into effect. I'm moving to Paris.

3

The Paris Plan

"We produce our lives like we produce a show" so many of my friends in TV said. And it was true. By summer 2015, The Paris Plan was in full swing. I had researched extensively. If I was going to leave everything I knew and everyone I loved, I wanted to have as much information as possible. I found an American University of Paris alum online and called them to see how their experience was. I watched YouTube videos and read the *Prêt à Voyager* blog obsessively, following the story of a woman named Anne who had made the leap many years before me.

I started free French classes at the French Church du Saint-Espirit in NYC and hired a tutor, a young American woman with a BA in French. I even bought a camera, a Canon DSLR, along with a microphone and mixer, to help me in my journalism endeavors abroad. It was pricey—I went with suggestions from my professional network—but at least I'd be ready to film at a moment's notice with a full camera kit.

I thought about The Paris Plan all the time: during a good day, a bad day, even while bored. I prayed about it, asking God to guide me to the right decision.

I sent off my application to AUP in June 2015 for September of the following year. I said my plans out loud often, to friends, to family, to anyone that would listen, as security that if I put it out into the universe, there was no backing down from it. Most responded with "Oh, really? That sounds nice." Doubt was written all over their faces. They didn't believe me—they thought it was a hoop dream. But many were supportive, including my first friend, my sister.

Although she was eight years older than me, we grew up close. Me tottering behind her all over the house, screaming and crying for our mom when she would close her bedroom door in my face. "Sometimes Crystal needs alone time," my mom would explain. I refused to be far from her, even sleeping in the bed together until our dad threatened to make my bedroom "the computer room" if I didn't use it. Effective way to get a six-year-old over her fear of sleeping alone.

Separate bedrooms didn't stop me from being obsessed with "Keiko," as I called her. I sat in the basement grinning like a Cheshire cat during her teenage sleepovers and bawled like a baby when my mother told me it was time for me to go to bed and leave the girls alone. What did she mean? I was one of the girls!

In her middle school woodworking class, she impressed her teachers by making a massive dollhouse for me, complete with vaulted ceilings and carpet. And when she left to attend Howard University, only a thirty-minute drive from home, I called her every day on her dorm room landline with one important question: "What did you eat for dinner today?"

We were close but wildly different. We both worked as journalists (her in newspapers and me in TV) and loved reading and writing—and the commonalities stopped there. I was more adventurous, an extrovert, and always on the go, compared to her homebody tendencies. She started traveling once I gifted her a trip to Europe using SkyMiles to get her out of her comfort zone. I was the one who always had a scheme, a proposal of some sort—a strategy. She wasn't surprised at all when I told her about The Paris Plan. She knew I was deeply unhappy with my current status at work, plus I had started traveling more, often taking two or three big trips a year with my friends.

She was a bit of a skeptic regarding the logistics of my plan, but she supported me. "What do you think Mom and Dad will say?" was her first question. Getting the support of my parents too would be a massive feat—near impossible. The only things they believed in more than Jesus were stability and family. I had a good job at a good company with good people—they wouldn't understand why I would leave. "Things happen in the Lord's time, not your time," my dad would say every time I bemoaned my lack of career advancement. "We do all things for the glory of the Lord, not man," he added. Job aside, they would wonder how I could live a life so far from our family unit.

In October 2015, a fat envelope with an American University of Paris seal arrived in the mail. I was ecstatic but kept the news to myself. I planned to break the news to my parents on Thanksgiving, when I returned from a South African vacation with my sister. As we were sitting in the airport in Cape Town, waiting for our flight back to the US, the airport TVs, all tuned to CNN, flashed a breaking news alert—there was some sort of kerfuffle at *Stade de France*, in Paris. Perhaps a bomb or maybe a stampede, they weren't sure. I grabbed my work phone, checking messages to see what was going on. Soon the news showed that it was more than something in the stadium—people were being gunned down in bars around the city and gunmen took hostages in a concert hall in an interconnected terrorist attack. The date was November 13, 2015.

As the days went on, the number of victims started to rise. Back at work, I produced news pieces about the attacks—repeatedly viewing disturbing security footage of gunmen in a restaurant, concertgoers jumping or falling from the Bataclan theater windows—bile rising in my throat. I started to reconsider The Paris Plan. I had lived in the DC area during 9/11, but aside from the Times Square bombing, my time in NYC had been relatively terrorism-free. The idea of moving to a place where I could be shot down enjoying a beer on a *terrasse* worried me. Ironic, considering the gun violence in America—I know.

I decided to forge ahead, sitting my parents down to inform them of my plan. I always wanted my parents' approval, despite my big age of thirty-one. Their support was important to me. My mind was made up, but I would feel more comfortable with their backing. Backing, as it turns out, that I wouldn't get.

"You want to move to *Paris?*" my dad asked in bewilderment. "Yes, that's the plan," I said, sliding the American University of Paris paperwork across the dining room table. My father took off his glasses and put his hand on his brow, his face screwed up in disbelief. My mother sat beside him, her lips poked out in disapproval. "Well, I'm going to pray that you meet a man so you won't go," my mother proclaimed.

It's funny—my expat dreams had been waylaid years earlier due to a man. The idea had previously crossed my mind to make the leap, and I found an MBA program in Spain. Spain was an obvious choice for me, having minored in Spanish at Howard—even though you couldn't tell after my years of neglect. I fretted over the application for months as I tried to muster up the courage to take a step toward a dream. But then, I met Brad.

Brad walked into my life that summer and changed it all for me. He wasn't my type—we met when I sat next to his best friend on a flight from Miami. A little bit of a "meet cute."

A former college football star, he worked in finance, and his style was more Vineyard Vines than the elevated streetwear I was used to. He wined and dined me, love-bombed me, and made plans for our future. He was a party animal (like many young NYC finance guys), but our chemistry was undeniable. He told me how I was better than any woman he'd met and that he wanted me to meet his mother. He added me on all of his social media accounts—Facebook, Instagram, even G-chat—something I never did unless things were serious. He flooded my email with links to elaborate vacations he wanted us to take, all on his dime.

He swept me up into a fairy tale—of course, there were compromises to be made on my side, but no one's perfect, right? For all of this, I had to get over that he often acted completely clueless about Black culture, despite being Black himself. "Ride or die? What does that mean?" At times I felt like the only Black person he knew—and I was certainly the only Black woman he'd ever dated. But no one's perfect, and I enjoyed spending time with him. Perhaps I'd found what I'd been looking for on my countless crazy New York City dates. Maybe dating outside of my type was all that it took.

I floated the idea of expat living to him one evening over pasta. "What do you think about living abroad? You like traveling, right?" I asked. "Yeah, I like traveling but I don't know about living out of the country," he replied. "Why not?" "I could never live that far from my mama," he countered not-so-jokingly. It was an answer I'd heard before on dates, but not from someone I wanted to take seriously. If I liked this guy and if we truly had the future that it seemed we did, maybe I owed it to myself to stick around and let it develop. Could I forgive myself if I'd been searching for love and found it, only to jet off to Madrid before it had a fighting chance? So that night, over my massive plate of pasta, I tucked the plan away in the back of my mind.

I closed the Madrid tabs on my browser and closed my

mind off to the plan. I released myself from skepticism and allowed myself to become vulnerable—soft—to open myself up to the possibility of a serious relationship with him. The application deadline passed without fanfare, and I settled on my decision.

Things were still going well with Brad. I'd recently splurged on his birthday gifts—gifts I was excited to give him. My love language was gifts and he always splurged on me, so why not return the favor? We didn't have plans on his actual birthday—he told me he wanted to go out with his boys, so I enjoyed a quiet night in, lying on my couch scrolling Instagram.

My thumb paused over an image, not quite sure what I was seeing. I squinted, trying to make sense of it, then bolted upright. Surely sitting up would solve the mystery of what I was seeing on Brad's Instagram account. I leaned over the phone, my heart caught in my throat. It was a blurry photo of Brad kissing a blonde woman—their eyes wild with excitement and a flurry of activity surrounding them. As I scrolled further, I realized it wasn't just that one picture, but several—and all posted a few minutes ago. I recognized his best friends and the bar where he said he would be celebrating his birthday. And just like that, it was over.

When I confronted him, he didn't deny it. He said he was out having fun and it just happened. He further explained that he thought it best that we break up because I wouldn't fit in with his friends. He was unwilling to explain more or even explain why, but I could read between the lines.

So there you have it. I gave up my dream and played

myself for a fool for a man who was more concerned about my race, complexion, hair type, and pedigree than who I truly am. And nothing hurts more than a man who isn't your type, someone you gave a chance to, playing you for a fool.

Fool me once.

My mother didn't know any of this. She had no idea that I'd toyed with the idea of moving abroad before or even that I had had a May–August romance that'd crushed my soul (yes, it was only three months but remember the love-bombing—not my fault). My mother's announcement that I must find someone was coincidental. But I'd been the fool before. I wouldn't be Boo Boo the Fool again. After her proclamation, I decided I simply wouldn't date until I landed on French soil. Can't be distracted by a man if you don't even allow yourself to look his way. Life is too short to let a man lead me astray again.

I would move forward with The Paris Plan no matter what.

◆ ◆ ◆

MY WINDOW AIR CONDITIONER UNITS noisily thrust out as much cool air as they could manage in the stifling August humidity. Boxes were everywhere. Stacked high in corners, lined up against the walls. A fine layer of cardboard dust mingled with dust bunnies on the floor. The day had come: I was leaving New York for Paris. I'd sold my couch and various hair appliances in advance of the big day, but it still seemed like the boxes kept multiplying.

Forty-eight hours earlier, I had walked out of Rockefeller Center for the last time, with a small tote bag full of my cubicle possessions accumulated over ten years. Twenty-four hours earlier, at my farewell party, I hugged the necks of friends who had become family. We danced and sang until the wee hours of the morning, capping the night off with Jay-Z songs—one about life in New York and one about life in Paris. Now my family was in my Harlem apartment, equal parts lugging my boxes and fussing at me for my lack of packing prowess.

As my family loaded the U-Haul to take my life in cardboard to their homes in Maryland, I leaned on the wall, looking out the window at the treetops of Central Park. So much had happened in this apartment—the apartment where I became a true adult, whether I felt it or not. The living room where I had hosted twenty-five women for a surprise bridal shower for my best friend, Traci—who conveniently lived right on my street.

The kitchen where I'd tried and failed on so many recipes, baked tons of brownies and cakes, and shared takeout and delivery meals with friends. The bedroom, my place of calm, at least until a mouse ran out from behind my dresser one night, leaving me a terrified and blubbering mess. I promptly called Traci, who sent her husband, Steve, over to talk me off the ledge—unsuccessfully. I ceded ownership of my apartment for the night and ended up sleeping on their couch.

Blinking back tears, I went from room to room—a two-minute tour, considering the apartment size. Was I making the right choice? So often in life you hear that if you're making the right decision, you'll never doubt it—you feel it instinctually. You're moving forward on the path you know was set for you. But here I was, tears rolling down my face as my anxiety ratcheted up notch by notch. If I still had so much fear, was I really doing the right thing? My silent tears turned to full-body racking sobs, to the alarm of my mother, who was always uncomfortable being within a ten-foot radius of crying.

"What's wrong? Why are you crying?" she asked, partly alarmed, partly uncomfortable, mostly concerned. "What-if-I'm-making-a-bad-decision?" I blurted in a sobbing gasp. "What-if-everything-goes-wrong?" "Well, you don't *have* to go," she said flippantly. "Or you can always come home," she suggested, a refrain that I would become well acquainted with over the next few years. It was simple but it was true. I could always come back.

It didn't immediately stop my tears, but it was a perspective I needed to remember. I wasn't a refugee—I wasn't running from war, human rights violations, or a toxic family. I wasn't going off with five dollars in my pocket, and I did have the support and network of the graduate program. I had made a choice to try to live life a little differently—and if it didn't work, I could go back to what I already knew. Which, for most people, wasn't that bad. But that didn't mean it wasn't still scary.

To my mother's delight, I stifled my sobs and straightened my back. Had my life in New York been the most amazing thing ever, or was I just afraid of leaving the familiar? I'd soon find out. My sister drove me to Newark airport on a ride that was comparable to a scene in the Fast and Furious movies as my parents' overloaded U-Haul lagged behind. I boarded my flight to Paris. I didn't know what was ahead of me—the rollercoaster I was boarding. How in less than two years, my life would turn upside down. I plopped into my seat on the plane. *On y va.*

• • •

LIFE IN PARIS WASN'T EVERYTHING I expected, even from the beginning. I moved to Paris to shake my life up, to make things interesting. I didn't realize that my move would be less of a tremor and more of a 9.0 Richter scale earthquake.

From the day I stepped off the plane at Charles de Gaulle Airport, things were different, much more different from what I thought they would be. Even with all of my research!

I arrived in Paris in August—the month known for its sweltering heat and lengthy French vacations. Stepping out of the airport into the wet heat, I had no idea it would be my last time feeling the cold blast of air conditioning for a while. If I had, I would have luxuriated in it more.

There were still signs of the November 2015 terrorist attack as well—police holding automatic rifles and military patrolling the streets. You'd even see them at the front of grocery stores, carrying assault weapons and inspecting bags before people could enter. It creeped me out—I understood the reasoning, but I also felt like I'd moved to a military state.

I had to hit the ground running once I arrived—I had to hustle and hustle *hard*. In addition to my master's program, I took all types of jobs, from teaching English to executives to managing an undergraduate editorial board to reading Diary of a Wimpy Kid books to a seven-year-old. Entitled but sweet, he once told me we needed to end our session early because his in-home masseuse had arrived for his appointment. It was a decent all-cash gig, other than constantly dodging his sixteen-year-old brother's lovestruck advances. He popped into our reading sessions with fake questions so often that his younger brother had to ask him to stop.

But the biggest unexpected difference? Living accommodations.

Before moving, I spent weeks scrolling Parisian real estate websites, looking at the gorgeous Haussmannian-style one-bedroom apartments for twelve hundred euros a month. The archways, the fireplaces, the crown molding, the French windows looking out onto a lush green *place*— *j'adore*. Online, the rent appeared to be cheaper than in NYC as well—the same thing would run you about two thousand dollars a month. I knew I wouldn't have any problems finding a decent place for a good price—there are so many Americans in Paris, *obviously* it can't be that hard. The lower cost of living was one of the major selling points of my move.

The university put me in temporary housing, in a dorm room with two other grad students, one from Chicago and the other from the Philippines. I was assured that I'd find a permanent home quickly—the school had its own database of apartments. To expedite the process, the school set me up with a partner, Laura, to help me find and visit apartments.

Looking at apartment after apartment with Laura left a lot to be desired. "You'll love this place, it's in a nice area," she said on our lengthy Métro ride. We arrived in the 14th arrondissement, walking fifteen minutes from the station to the studio apartment. It was well decorated but small—one narrow room with a sofa bed and specks of mold in the corners. The apartment needed a good paint job.

The landlord busied herself, running from corner to corner—giving a tour as if we were in the *Château de Versailles* and not an apartment the size of a one-car garage. From the rusty hot plate to the minuscule bathroom I could barely turn around in. "Not for me," I told my partner after we stepped outside.

We trudged over to the second apartment on the list—walking distance from the school and only a few blocks from the Eiffel Tower. The landlord was a good one, she assured me, because they rented to students often. But the apartment was more well suited for a child's playhouse than a home for your average-sized university student. I crouched beneath the low ceiling—I could barely stand up at my entire five-foot-four height. Laura, who was much taller, tried to convince me it was normal and that I should go ahead and sign.

It was depressing and confusing. Everything was so different from what I expected—so much smaller, moldier, and much more expensive. Where were the beautiful one-bedroom apartments for twelve hundred euros that I had seen online? Where was the crown molding? Where were the French windows even? Every apartment we entered, Laura would say encouragingly, "Well, this one seems nice; see, the hot plate looks new!" My face would fall into a scowl. As they say in the South, please don't pee on my head and tell me it's raining.

I wasn't picky, but every apartment had "suitable for a twenty-two-year-old who has never lived outside of a dorm before" written all over it. At thirty-two years old, what could I do with these tiny, dank, and limiting apartments? A hot plate? A sofa bed? Everything looked decrepit or like it was made for the very petite. I had left my sunny one-bedroom apartment in Harlem for this? I was ready to make sacrifices, but I wasn't willing to let my quality of life fall that far.

After several depressing visits, pressured to sign for apartments where I knew I would be unhappy, I took matters into my own hands. It helped, of course, that the university was threatening to kick me out of the temporary housing.

I visited a tiny studio via an expat agency in the 6th arrondissement, in the chic neighborhood of Saint-Germain. It was a few streets over from *Café de Flore* and *Les Deux Magots*, restaurants frequented by Ernest Hemingway, Pablo Picasso, and James Baldwin. Even better, the apartment was on *Rue Princesse*. I took it as a sign that I was setting myself up for success.

Never mind that *Rue Princesse* was jam-packed with Irish, British, and American pubs. It was only fifteen minutes by bus from school, the building and street looked well taken care of and clean, and it fit my budget. I signed on the dotted line—for nine hundred sixty-five euros a month plus utilities and renter's insurance, I rented an apartment the size of an American parking space. I had to pay six months' rent in advance due to my student status and vowed to invest in earplugs. It wasn't the apartment I had dreamed of when I sat in my sunny one-bedroom in Harlem—*pas de tout*. But at least I had a permanent place. Or so I thought.

A battered sofa served as the main piece of furniture in the room. It was the bed, it was the lounger, it was everything. There was a small two-person table across from the sofa—if the sofa was extended into a bed, I couldn't use the table. So every morning I put my bed away. The kitchen was one foot from the bed and the bathroom was two steps from the kitchen, if that. The best part? The water heater was above the toilet, so you had to cautiously get up from the toilet seat or you could find yourself knocked unconscious, crumpled in a heap on the bathroom floor (because of course it's too small for you to fall in a prone position).

A ten-inch TV was mounted on a wall, so at least you could watch TV while you cook . . . while you lie in bed . . . while you're on the toilet. That is, if the TV worked. But I had my laptop and iPad so I figured that would be fine—until I was unable to get internet. The service provider said it was *"c'est pas possible"* (a phrase I'd come to hear all the time) to have internet unless I gave them the name and number of the person who lived in the apartment before me. I didn't know and neither did the owners, so that was the end of that. I called and called internet providers, even showing up tearfully in person one day with a French-speaking Tinder date. After he failed to move the process along, I gave up.

Every day, I squeezed my way around the tiny apartment, opening the sofa bed before sleeping and closing it in the mornings. The lack of internet was not ideal for a grad student. I spent the majority of my time after school at a nearby Starbucks, which was open until 11 p.m. I would grab a drink and sit on the top floor, doing my homework surrounded by other students, tourists, and occasionally the unhoused. When Starbucks kicked me out for the night, I'd go to eat ramen at Ippudo—they closed at 1 a.m. I would be home by 1:30 a.m., pulling out my sofa bed to go to sleep and start it all over again.

My family came to visit me after two months in Paris. As they looked around the tiny place, their faces fought to not show their opinions on my new home. To be fair, my apartment was larger than some of my classmates' apartments, but I was also much older than most of them. I stayed in the apartment for four months, too tired to begin my search again in earnest and also too busy with the crushing workload of grad school. I understood making sacrifices for a new life, but I wanted to be comfortable enough to stay long term. This apartment was the beginning of my apartment woes—one that would become a pattern in my new life in Paris.

4

Testing, Testing

Shell-shocked after my gynecology appointment with Dr. Boucher, I launched myself into a whirlwind adventure in the French medical system. And what a whirlwind adventure it was.

For two weeks, they poked, prodded, and tested me like a lab rat. My doctor wrote prescriptions for tests I couldn't pronounce in French—tests I didn't know how to book appointments for in France. I googled but wasn't sure what to google for. I called medical imaging offices, asking in my stilted French, *"Parlez-vous anglais?"* Thankfully, they often responded *"oui"* or *"un petit peu,"* which meant they had enough English to get by in our conversation.

It was scary—I didn't know if I was doing anything right—and as a matter of fact, I was sure I wasn't. Everything moved so fast, but the breakneck speed of going from test to test helped keep my mind off of things. I had something to do, tasks to complete. If I followed all the steps and did all the tests, perhaps it all would work out in the end. Do the tests, get the benign result. Nothing more to it.

First up: the mammogram and MRI. Dr. Boucher recommended a place near the famed *Champs-Elysées*, and it resembled more of a spa than a medical facility. I had had MRIs before, but only in the US, where I knew what to expect. I ducked into the well-appointed office, gripping my *ordonnance*—prescription—that my doctor had written for the test. A chandelier glittered over a spiral staircase; leather couches lined the reception area. A blonde woman with a tight topknot capped off the spa vibes. I approached the desk and handed her my papers. "Carte Vitale?" she said without looking up at me.

The famous *Carte Vitale*. The *Carte Vitale* is a green card given by the French government to citizens and residents in France—even those studying in France for over three months. The card is, as the literal translation suggests, essential for all healthcare in France and is linked with an online account and your bank account. It gives you access to France's healthcare system, which is famously low priced (but not free) and subsidized via taxpayer money.

Unfortunately, I didn't have one. Despite living in France for two years, my school didn't apply for the *Carte Vitale* for grad students over the age of twenty-six. And no, I have no clue what their reasoning was—maybe just another way to make me feel old. I paid for private insurance through the university, which helped. Thankfully, with my new job, they applied for the card for me, but as I'd only started a month earlier, I didn't have it yet.

"Je n'ai pas une Carte Vitale," I told her, not knowing it would be a phrase I would repeat endlessly. She huffed at my response, knowing without the *Carte Vitale*, there would be more paperwork on her end. She shoved papers across the desk toward me, including a bill. "Okay, well, you pay this now, before your appointment," she said, annoyed with my strong American-accented French and switching to English.

I looked down, not expecting to see a bill of five hundred euros on the table. "All of it? Right now?" I ran a quick calculation in my head. Taking this job, while it was something I wanted, was a massive pay cut from my previous job in NYC—about a sixty percent pay cut. Not to mention I didn't work full-time while completing my master's degree and wasn't taking home much after France's notoriously high taxes. I reached into my bag and handed over my American Express. "We don't take American Express, *Madame*, only Visa," she informed me. With a wince and a sigh, I handed over my debit card.

Each appointment was more of the same. Me arriving and nervously speaking to them in my stilted French, them hearing my accent and switching to English. It annoyed me every time—I was making the effort to improve my French, but the opportunity was always taken from me. And then, of course, the dreaded *Carte Vitale* conversation. My mammogram: "Two hundred euros, *Madame*; we don't take American Express."

My final test was the guided biopsy. "One hundred fifty euros, no American Express, but don't worry, you'll get reimbursed," the receptionist explained. A guided biopsy is a painful procedure where a needle, guided by a sonogram, takes breast tissue from the lump for testing. I handed over my Visa again, trying not to grimace. "Okay, you'll get your results in about two weeks," the receptionist said, handing my card back to me.

"Two weeks? Is it possible to get it sooner?"

"No, two weeks is the average. Your doctor will call you to make an appointment for the results."

I plodded out of the office, stunned. How could I be expected to wait two weeks for such life-altering news? Wasn't the point of doing this battery of testing to get comprehensive results more quickly? Two weeks would feel like a lifetime.

I couldn't stop comparing my journey to what it would be back home. Despite the tests being cheaper than they would be in America, I was quickly running out of money. The reimbursements from my private insurance wouldn't arrive for six weeks or more.

When I told friends back home about my situation, everyone said, "You're so lucky you're in France, where you have free healthcare." It's true that I was lucky to be in France, but not true that the healthcare was free. The cost was much lower but still a strain on my finances, especially when you're undergoing expensive tests back-to-back. But I wasn't allowed to say that—so I smiled and nodded, while praying for my bank account not to overdraft.

The speed with which I was able to get my tests done was a silver lining. I didn't have the common insurance delays like in the US. I wasn't waiting for my insurance to green-light the tests or send me to a specific in-network provider. But the truth was, I was still adjusting to a monthly paycheck (as opposed to the biweekly schedule I was used to) and the significant pay cut. My finances felt the strain. I yearned for the ability to put down a co-pay of fifty to one hundred euros and figure out the rest once the bill came in the mail.

The US was the only point of reference I had. I didn't know anyone who had been through a cancer scare in France—or abroad, period. I fired up Google, searching for how long biopsy results would take in the US. How different could this journey be if I closed up shop and flew back home? Well, at the very least, Google told me, my biopsy results would only take forty-eight to seventy-two hours. Had I made a mistake? Even if I had, it was too late. Self-doubt plagued me morning, noon, and night.

However, unlike in the US, after every imaging test, I was sent home with the images to keep. It was an unexpected perk, but it also added more to my anxiety. Late at night, kept awake by my worries, I would pull out my sonogram and MRI slides, trying to self-diagnose.

The two weeks were hell. Absolute hell. I went to work as normal, welcoming the distraction from my looming test results. After work, I walked across the street to my apartment, a bizarrely laid-out place with steep art deco–style stairs leading to a lofted bed—the bed squeezed under the sloped ceiling. I crouched around the apartment after work, changing clothes and then setting off into the Parisian streets.

And then I walked. I walked and walked and walked. I would walk the city from 7 p.m. to nearly 2 or 3 a.m. I walked from my apartment in the western reaches of the 16th arrondissement to *Hôtel de Ville*—City Hall—in the center of Paris, in the 1st.

I rarely stopped to eat or drink. I had no appetite to speak of. I just walked and walked, looking at everything around me but barely taking it in. I peeked into secret courtyards hidden behind massive doors, when people walked into their apartment buildings at night. I saw university students spilling into and out of bars and the unhoused making their beds for the night. I saw the sky turn pink as the sun set over the Seine and the city descended into darkness.

I've always been a walker. Talk to my family and they'll recount several stories from my childhood when I got in trouble for wandering off and convincing my friends, "It's not too far—we can walk there." It even earned me the familial nickname of "Legs." I enjoy walking—it's one of the many reasons I love living in cities—but it's less about the exercise and more about the distraction.

Walking is a form of meditation for me. Walking the city, I wasn't so focused on the test results. They were still on my mind, sure, but I was distracted. One foot in front of the other—each step felt like I was reducing my hellish wait time. I tried to focus on the beauty around me, seeing the city I gave up so much to live in. The City of Light, the City of Love. It felt like neither for me—it felt like I had blown up my life. Was my situation—the possible cancer diagnosis—because of my move to Paris or in spite of it?

And so I walked. If things were going to go to hell in a handbasket, I should make sure I saw enough of the city I sacrificed so much to be in. I paused to watch street performers: an old man on an accordion (honestly, I thought it was simply a trope before I moved to Paris—who knew?), a group of teens breakdancing. I stopped on bridges, waving back to the tourists on the *Bateau-Mouche* crossing underneath, remembering over twenty years earlier when I was on the boat just like them. Sometimes I whispered a little prayer to myself, asking God that the scare would be just that—a scare. It was time to call in my favors with God, time to pay the piper. I hoped he heard me.

Once my feet tired and sleep was imminent (I hoped), I returned to my sixth-floor apartment and collapsed on the couch. No use climbing the steep stairs to the bed like a spider monkey if I didn't have to. I lay on the couch, tossing and turning, hoping for sleep that rarely came. I woke up at 8 a.m. to face another workday and start the whole thing over again.

Wash, rinse, repeat.

• • •

"MADEMOISELLE." AN ENORMOUS GLASS OF rosé, the pale pink wine shimmering in the sunlight, landed on my table. After a two-week wait, I would finally get my answer. It was a beautiful late-June day—the sun shining bright and tourists crawling all over the city. I watched from the *terrasse* as families with fanny packs and cameras around their necks walked toward the Eiffel Tower.

Today was the big day. My stomach roiled. Wringing my hands, I attempted to calm myself in the *brasserie* a few streets from my doctor's office. Thankfully, I wasn't alone. My friend Lyneka came with me—her mother had beat breast cancer several years earlier. She offered to join to celebrate what we hoped would be the news that my lump was benign.

"How are you feeling; are you good?" she asked, joining me at my table. I took a swig of my wine—I wasn't there to savor the taste. "I think it'll be okay, but I am nervous," I admitted.

Lyneka was my closest friend in Paris. We had both majored in journalism at Howard but only met after graduating, once we both moved to NYC. She moved to Paris about a year before me and she, along with my friend Nicole from my graduate program, were my closest confidants. Unfortunately, like most of the people in my graduate program, Nicole had left a few months earlier to move back to Canada. I needed all the support I could get, and I was so happy to have Lyneka with me.

I chugged the wine to completion and headed over to Dr. Boucher's office. Let's end this nightmare.

Plopping into the chair opposite Dr. Boucher, my friend

by my side, I was still hopeful. Hopeful this was all some sort of mix-up, some sort of bad dream. Hopeful that maybe I had eaten too many almonds and we would laugh it off and I could change my diet. Hopeful this would just be a blip in my Paris story. The hope was short-lived.

"So," she began in her French-accented English, after our pleasantries, "we ran all of the tests. And the tumor is malignant."

I blinked. I gazed at her silently, my face a stone wall. Maybe I didn't hear her correctly—or maybe she hadn't actually spoken at all. I blinked again. I opened my mouth but couldn't speak. The walls of hope I'd built up around me began to crack, crumble, and fall away one by one. The walls were gone, and I was unprotected. My stomach lurched as if I was falling, but I still clung to a morsel of hope.

"So it's cancerous?" I asked, my last-ditch effort to see the situation clearly.

Dr. Boucher leaned forward, her expression grim. "It's cancerous. It's called DCIS, which is a cancer that goes in the milk ducts." I felt Lyneka stiffen in the chair next to me. I couldn't look at her—that would make the whole situation too real. I could only look straight ahead or at my hands, still clasped tightly in my lap.

That's it. The hope was gone, even the tiny bit I had left. DCIS, ductal carcinoma in situ, she explained, means that the cancer has not spread to any of the other breast tissue. Dr. Boucher went on, explaining it was one of the "best possible breast cancers."

She scheduled an appointment for me in two days with a friend of hers, an excellent cancer surgeon at the American Hospital. It was easier—and possibly faster—for me to go through the private system, she said, since I didn't have my *Carte Vitale* yet.

As she droned on about next steps, I sat in stunned silence. I felt as if I had blacked out—she made as much sense to me as the garbled words of Charlie Brown's teacher. The world and time were suspended as I tried and failed to process the shocking news.

"When you call your parents, make sure you tell them you have the best possible breast cancer," she said, bringing my attention back to the present. I forgot about having to tell my family. My family, who was currently away in New Orleans for a conference, anxiously waiting for an update but convinced their fervent prayers had worked. After all, it's not like we had any family history of breast cancer.

"My daughter, she lives in Boston," she said. My eyes glanced over to the photo on her mantel showing a pretty brown-haired woman in a graduation cap and gown. My doctor stood next to her, their smiles identical. "It would be scary for me to get news like that about her from so far away. So make sure you tell them that. It'll be okay," she said.

We stood to leave, both me and Lyneka in a shell-shocked state. Dr. Boucher embraced me, an extremely rare gesture in France. While hugging my doctor, the gravity of the situation began to set in. That was the first indication I was going up against something serious. A French person hugging you, unprompted—clearly the situation is not okay.

We separated from the embrace, her assuring me all would be well. "Is there anything else you need from me before you go?" she asked.

All my sleepless nights of wandering the city came back to me in a flash. "I need some Xanax!"

I left the office still feeling stunned, Xanax prescription in my hand. My elevator, the one that felt like it was going up a couple of weeks ago, halted. Someone had pushed the emergency stop button, and I had no idea when it would start moving again.

5

Life Comes at You Fast and So Does Cancer

We left the gynecologist's office in shock. I hadn't expected the diagnosis—after all, I had no family history of breast cancer. I drank, but I never drank too much. I tried to eat well and I exercised. I tried to be a good person—I prayed, went to church, and respected my parents. I was only thirty-four. All the risk factors for breast cancer didn't apply. These things didn't happen to me or people like me. At least, that's what I thought.

When Dr. Boucher said those dreaded words, "You have cancer," I knew my life was going to change. But I had no idea how much. My agency over my own body, my own health, seemed to vanish overnight as I was assaulted with test after test. And it would probably be worse once I started all my treatments, whatever they would be.

I floated through the streets of Paris, for once not taking

in the sights around me. I realized I had to tell my family. They were awaiting my news—expecting good news, so we could all move on from this small scare of when we thought Robin might have cancer. I called my mother, forcing lightness into my voice. "Hey, Robin," my mother answered, the buzz of conversation and coffee machines whirring in the background. "I'm in Starbucks; your dad is getting the drinks. Did you hear from the doctor?" I stood on a quiet side street, gazing up at the ornate buildings of the 7th arrondissement.

What kind of lives do the people living in these luxury buildings have? Did they ever have to go through this?

It would be my first time saying it out loud—I wanted to get it over with. I inhaled deeply.

"I did—so I have cancer. But! The doctor says it's the best possible breast cancer to have." The words rushed out with a false chirp in my voice. *"What!"* my mom exclaimed, horrifying everyone in the New Orleans Starbucks. I imagined jolted caramel macchiatos burning fingers and college students popping their heads up over their MacBooks.

"She said it's going to be okay. I have an appointment with a surgeon this week and—" "A surgeon?" She cut me off, her voice wavering. The more I spoke, the worse it was going. I'd never seen my mother cry before—remember, she was uncomfortable with tears—but I was certain tears were falling on the other end of the phone.

My father's voice came onto the phone in a panic. "Robin, what happened?" I could hear my mother attempting to explain, too upset to fully relay the story. Why I decided to tell them such life-changing news in a Canal

Street Starbucks, I'll never know. But I do know, as I listened to the muffled pandemonium on the other end of the phone, I regretted my lack of foresight. I began to feel worse and worse.

"The doctor said I have breast cancer," I repeated, nervous about breaking the news for a second time in Starbucks. "Really?" my dad replied. "Okay, well, listen, I have to get your mother out of here." My mom's sniffles were still audible in the background. "We'll go back to the hotel and call you back from there." We disconnected, and I stared at the dark phone in my hand.

Still numb with shock from the dramatic events of the last hour, for the first time, sadness hit me. But not just sadness—I felt guilty. I'd devastated my parents with the news and probably caused a minor disruption in a New Orleans Starbucks.

Over the last few years of my life in the US, receiving panicked early morning and late-night phone calls was a regular occurrence. I would awaken out of my slumber to my closest friends wailing on the line, having lost a parent suddenly. I would throw on clothes and head over immediately to help comfort my friend in any way I could. After so many of these calls, I dreaded answering late-night and early morning calls, hoping it wasn't more news of a lost loved one. I worried that one day I'd receive a similar call from my sister, about my own parents. I never expected that one day, the bad news could be me.

◆ ◆ ◆

I WAS WALKING THROUGH LIFE like a zombie. My diagnosis hit me in the face like a brick—I stumbled around blinded by the pain, racked with confusion about why it had happened to me. Thanks to Xanax, I was sleeping at night, but I was still on edge during my waking hours.

My mother always talked about seeing women crying in the streets of Paris whenever she visited—she found it to be a bizarre phenomenon. Well, it was my turn to take part: I cried and cried often. I cried walking to work and cried walking home from work. I cried in the grocery store. I cried whenever I thought too hard about my unknown future. Life felt like a cruel joke.

Following Dr. Boucher's orders, I made my first trip to the American Hospital in Neuilly-sur-Seine. Wide, tree-lined streets led to the renowned hospital, located in a monied suburban neighborhood. Massive stone apartment buildings with iron balconies were set back from the sidewalk, gates closed to keep out the riffraff. There were even large single-family homes with circular driveways—a sight not commonly seen in Paris proper. Children were pushed in strollers by women with no familial resemblance. You couldn't find trash on the streets or even an errant cigarette stub. It's a suburb of Paris accessible by a thirty-minute Métro ride, but in many ways, it felt like a different world.

The American Hospital of Paris wasn't your normal hospital by a long shot. It was known for being one of the most expensive hospitals in Paris—many of the doctors didn't take *Carte Vitale*, which meant patients were paying out of pocket or insured in other ways. If they did take *Carte Vitale*, their prices were still far above what the French system would reimburse. Because of this, the hospital was mostly used by expats, foreigners, and the French upper echelon. Nearly a third of all patients were foreign, flying in from Africa, the Middle East, and all over the world to receive quality care.

And that's not to say the French public system didn't provide quality care—to the contrary. The care was world-class in France, whether you decided to go public or private. But for those of us outside the *Carte Vitale* system, the private system had fewer hoops to jump through for urgent situations, even though it was more expensive.

Walking in, I didn't feel like I was in a hospital at all. You didn't hear the normal beeps and alarms, only the cheery *"bonjours"* of staff and soft shoes on the carpet-lined hallways. The hustle and bustle of normal hospitals didn't seem to exist there. No overwhelming smell of antiseptic.

Outside, Rolls-Royces and Mercedes-Benzes dropped off their well-heeled passengers. A valet stood at the ready to take your car—and could even provide car-washing services, if needed. It reminded me more of a hotel than a hospital, which reassured me, for better or worse. A hotel, I can handle. A hospital, not so much.

Despite the obviously monied people around me, I didn't feel out of place. There were young families and people bringing their grandparents in. The patients were diverse in age, ethnicity, and nationality. Even with "American" in the name of the hospital, the language barrier was still present. It functioned like a French hospital—everything was done in French and everyone employed was French.

Many of the doctors also spoke English, but I often needed to rely on my broken French for administrative matters. I arrived with Lyneka for my appointment with the oncology surgeon. Firm blue couches lined the waiting room, packed with women, all waiting for their fifteen minutes in the sun—the one-hundred-and-fifty-euro consultation with Dr. Toussaint, the surgeon with the gifted hands.

We sat on the polyester couch, not knowing what to expect. We waited for ten minutes. Fifteen. Thirty. Forty-five. An hour-long wait, watching the revolving door of women parade in and out of the office. Women of all ages and races and sizes, women with their spouses, women with their children, women who were pregnant—some left the office happy, some with grim expressions, some with unreadable faces. I appeared to be the youngest one there.

"*Madame* Davis!" The soft-spoken baritone snapped me out of my fog and into the present. Dr. Toussaint was ready for me, but I'm not sure I was ready for him. I expected a short white man with a shock of gray hair—maybe I'd watched too many movies. A tall man with a head full of dark hair greeted me in his office. He easily could have been an airline pilot—he had the look. He moved with confidence and ease and wore his tailored blue suit well. He had a cool air about him, as if he could fly through a tornado and wouldn't be rattled. He could turn on the in-flight announcement system and calm passengers' nerves with his soft baritone.

"I received your file from Dr. Boucher," he started, after we sat down and exchanged pleasantries. "What I'm recommending is a single mastectomy with immediate reconstruction, and we should do it as soon as possible." Way to jump right into it. I was still admiring his office, particularly the picture window behind him with a view of the lush greenery of the courtyard. Lyneka had brought a notepad, remembering how I seemingly blacked out during the last appointment. I heard the scribble of her furious note-taking next to me, her pencil loudly scratching the paper.

"Wait—but if I have the 'good' cancer, why do I have to have a mastectomy? Why can't I have a lumpectomy?"

"Well, it all depends on the size of the lump. Your lump measures six centimeters—about the size of an egg—which is too large for a lumpectomy." He grabbed a piece of paper on his desk and began to draw a breast. "You see, you have DCIS, which means the cancer is in the milk ducts." He drew a large circle with ridges, to represent the alien form inside my chest. It looked like one of those drawings that cold and flu medicines use in their commercials to represent germs.

"And this is your lump," he said, pointing to the ridged circle. "Yes, but I thought DCIS meant it's more contained than other types of breast cancer," I said. "Well, in order to take it out and have clear margins—which is the amount of space needed between the cancerous tissue and healthy tissue—you have to take a large amount of the breast," he explained. He drew an X to show the amount of surgery required. Lyneka and I both leaned forward in our chairs, inspecting his artwork.

"But—so—you have to do a mastectomy? There's no

way around it?" I asked, desperation creeping into my voice. "Yes," he replied definitively, nodding his head. "Well, if that's the case I want a double mastectomy. Take both," I declared.

It sounded like a quick decision, but it wasn't. I'd heard of women having a double mastectomy for cancer and if I *had* to lose a breast, I'd rather lose both, so I wouldn't spend the rest of my life worrying about the other. A double mastectomy would hopefully free me of any future worries and probably give a better aesthetic result as a silver lining.

"No, we won't do that," he said. Lyneka and I stared at him, mouths agape.

"If I have it in one breast, I don't want to worry about it coming back in another breast, so why can't I get both?"

"It doesn't skip from breast to breast, so you don't have to worry about that." I mused over this information as Lyneka continued to go to bat for me.

His refusal shocked me. It seemed bizarre that I wouldn't be allowed to get a double—after all, it was *my* body, so it should be *my* choice. But at that moment, it didn't feel that way. The loss of agency over my body was overwhelming. My mind wouldn't stop going back to how things would be in the US—a request like mine wouldn't immediately be rejected, and if I fought hard enough, I'm sure it would be granted.

Maybe, I mused, I should just trust what everyone tells me—especially in a foreign country that perhaps handles cancer in a different way than my homeland. Different, but would it be better? How would I know? I'd never had cancer before. It was decided, whether I liked it or not, I wouldn't have a double mastectomy.

Dr. Toussaint explained how the surgery would work: He would work in tandem with a plastic surgeon. He would operate first, removing the tumor and several of my lymph nodes to see if the cancer had spread. He would then test the tumor and lymph nodes—it would be the determining factor for whether I needed chemotherapy or radiation. He explained that the plastic surgeon, Dr. Gauthier, would then lift my pectoral muscle from the chest wall and put an implant underneath. Surgery would be in two weeks.

"July twelfth?" I asked as Lyneka scribbled the date into her notebook. "Do you have family in France that can come to be with you?" he responded.

"Yes," I said. "My family will figure something out."

"Or if not, I will be there with her," Lyneka offered. I looked over at Lyneka gratefully, glancing at the notebook she brought with her. The pages were full of scrawl—diligent journalist that she is, she took pages and pages of notes for me. She knew I would barely remember any details once we walked out of the office. By the end of the ordeal, she'd have enough pages to publish a book, *The Sad State of Affairs of Robin's Breasts (Vol. 1)*.

He took me to a tiny room adjacent to his office for an exam. I still wasn't used to being topless around male doctors without a female nurse present—but I was sure by the end of this I would be. After the exam, across from his massive cherry oak L-shaped desk, we mused about the cause of the cancer. "Do we know what could have caused it?" Lyneka asked.

"It could be anything. It could be genetic; it could be environmental. We don't know, and it's possible we may never know. These things happen," Dr. Toussaint said.

"So is there anything Robin shouldn't eat or drink or do before the surgery?" she asked, her pencil racing across her notebook pages. "No, everything is fine, she can do what she wants," he said. "What about alcohol, wine . . . ?" Dr. Toussaint smiled.

"It's France—you must drink the wine," he said with a laugh.

If that wasn't the Frenchest thing I'd ever heard.

We left the hospital with folders full of documents—appointments made with the anesthesiologists and plastic surgeon, phone numbers to call in my tote bag. Back on the tree-lined streets of Neuilly-sur-Seine, I called my parents during the long walk to the Métro. "How did you like the surgeon?" my family asked. "I liked him—he drew a picture!" It's funny what sticks out the most in your mind.

Everything was moving faster than I expected. Talking to my parents, they floated the idea of going back to the US for treatment. "You know you can always come back," they offered.

There goes that line again—and it was true, I could always go back. But I had no health insurance in the US. Health insurance was linked to having a job in the US, which I didn't have. Even if I could get on Medicaid, how quickly could that happen? How would I pay for a mastectomy in the US—forget the mastectomy, paying for all the tests leading up to the mastectomy would likely bankrupt me first.

In theory, I was covered by the French national insurance even without receiving my *Carte Vitale* to put things into motion. I emailed human resources at my workplace to see if they could expedite the card. "I have a few medical things coming up. Is there a way I can get the card sooner?" I pleaded. "Sorry, no, that's not possible. Delay until you get the card," the HR official responded. It's not her fault—she didn't know what she was asking me to delay was a life-saving operation.

No one at work knew I was diagnosed with cancer—I kept it a secret out of fear of job termination. I'd only officially been working there less than two months before my diagnosis. If I told them and ended up losing my job, I would have even bigger problems, considering my job was sponsoring my residency—my right to live—in France.

I felt helpless, trapped between two systems, both of which were not entirely ideal. The tests in France put a strain on me financially, but they were pennies compared to how much it would be in the US, especially without insurance. Now there was an added sense of urgency, since my doctor wanted to operate almost immediately. If he wanted to operate so soon, did that mean my cancer could spread quickly? Would I survive the back-and-forth, paperwork shuffle delay of moving back to the US for treatment?

Thankfully, I still had a few more months of coverage left on the AUP private health insurance. If everything had to be done quickly, at least there was a chance everything could be covered under that policy. Staying in France would be the best move for me—and I just had to hope I was making the right decision.

◆ ◆ ◆

IN THE PAST, TRAVEL HAD always sustained me. Whenever life felt too hard or I needed time and space to sort my thoughts, going somewhere new always helped. And when I couldn't afford to travel, I went somewhere familiar I could rediscover—like my weekly Central Park walks.

When I had arrived in Paris two years ago, in August 2016, it was hot. It was hot and sticky, and I'd never been so sweaty in my life. I couldn't sleep at night in the sweltering heat; my deodorant struggled to work in the muggy weather. I found myself sniffing my armpits and being horrified to discover the funk came from me.

It didn't matter that I'd experienced higher temps before—it was in the nineties—but what did matter was the lack of strong air conditioning. The heat was relentless, without any breaks. I'd been in Paris for a week and I found myself ducking into Starbucks and Picard, the frozen food store, for a blast of cool air.

After moving into my grandiose hovel in Saint-Germain, fighting (and failing) to get internet access, I decided I needed a trip. I booted up my laptop at Starbucks and researched where I could go quickly and cheaply—and landed on Brussels. I'd never been there, and it was only a five-hour bus ride: doable for both my grad student budget and schedule.

I logged into the Hilton website and, using a portion of the thousands of points I'd accrued from work travel, booked a hotel room—*with* air conditioning, of course. I was going to sleep in a bed that didn't have to be folded. I was going to sleep without sweating through the sheets. I was going to live like a queen for a weekend in a little Hilton Garden Inn in Brussels. And I did.

Ever since then, whenever I needed a break or a reset, I headed to the Hilton Garden Inn in Brussels. Sometimes, I didn't even leave the hotel room apart from grabbing some food. There was a tiny bodega across the street along with a Domino's. I would rest, eat pizza, watch TV, and journal. Sometimes, I met up with friends in the city or did a walking tour, taking in sights such as the Grand Plaza and the peeing child statue, *Manneken Pis,* and going to Delirium for world-famous Belgian beer. But mostly, I would rest.

Brussels became one of my favorite getaways. One perk of moving to Paris was the ease of travel throughout Europe, and it certainly delivered. I went to Brussels whenever I had the time or an extra fifty euros to spend on the bus—or a hundred and fifty euros to spend on the Thalys train.

Soon, I was able to walk the city and take transport without needing to check my phone for directions. I was able to practice my French—the Belgians were much kinder about my status as a French learner than the Parisians were. And if my French failed me, many people in Brussels spoke English due to the various international organizations headquartered there, like NATO. I loved Brussels. It was like a calmer, colder, and friendlier Paris. With more beer.

My surgery date was looming. I met the plastic surgeon, yet another man I took my top off for. It was starting to feel routine, and I'd learned to make sure I wore a blouse to all my appointments, as opposed to a dress. I wanted to get away and feel like myself again. Forget about surgery, breasts, everything. Maybe dance on top of a bar or flirt with a cute guy. Maybe shop or laugh until I cried. I needed something different before my life irreparably changed. I craved excitement—the good kind. I'd had too much of the bad kind. So I booked a trip to London.

Before moving to Paris, I wasn't too fond of London, but I'd grown to appreciate the city since my move. Being in London felt almost like home—the language barrier was nonexistent and the city buzzed with a familiar energy. I understood more of the cultural norms in London than in Paris. Every trip, I brought an empty suitcase to load up with hair products—from deep conditioners to crochet hair—because the selection was better in London. I could stop at a Jamaican restaurant to order a beef patty, jerk chicken, or both—it was one of my favorite cuisines, nearly impossible to find in Paris.

I exhaled loudly as I stepped off the train into London's St. Pancras station. It was my last weekend to live it up, last weekend to be a woman with two breasts, last weekend to live life not marked as the "woman who had breast cancer." A breast cancer survivor. I shuddered at the thought. The clipped and lilting tones of British English greeted me—pleasing to my ears. I wasn't home, but I was close enough.

I wandered the streets of East London, my favorite

neighborhood, eating from as many of the food stands as I could in the Spitalfields Market. I marveled at all the various cuisines, snapping photos to reminisce on later. I photographed street art, pausing to reflect on a massive mural of a dark-skinned Black woman with locs, gazing at the sky.

In Notting Hill, I chuckled at all the Harry and Meghan tchotchkes for sale, from their wedding two months prior. I bought a magnet of the beaming couple to place ironically on my refrigerator. I stumbled across a street market, browsing the artisanal offerings, and ducked into the famed Notting Hill bookstore, still cashing in on their movie fame from decades earlier.

I even went to the hair salon: my favorite stylist was based in London. One thing about me—possibly about all Black women—when my hair is done, I feel invincible. My hair was not only my crown but also my armor. It didn't matter that I had an appointment to get my hair braided for surgery four days later. She whipped my hair into shape, massaging my scalp, conditioning my hair, and trimming my ends. When your stylist is gifted, there's nothing more luxurious than a hair appointment.

I engaged in shoptalk—something I missed in Paris. I asked the women what they thought of their new Duchess Meghan, then laughed as the salon erupted into a fierce debate. I stepped out of the salon feeling like a million dollars, my hair whipping in the London breeze. The cut and silk press gave me wings. My crown was polished. I could soar above it all, I could beat the cancer, I could go through surgery like it was nothing. All while feeling and looking fly.

I took the Tube to South London to eat the Jamaican food I so missed in Paris, gorging myself at an outdoor table at the tiny Jamaican restaurant in Brixton Market. When the steaming plate of jerk chicken arrived at my table, I could have cried. The spice, the flavors, the vibes—I was in heaven.

I strolled the market. The stores were a mix of clothing, Colombian food, West African home goods, and artisanal wares. I went to almost every stall, touching the fabrics, chatting with the shop owners. I stopped in another restaurant—ordering padrón peppers, a dish I loved in NYC. When the waitress stopped by to check on me, a mere few minutes later, she gaped at the empty bowl in front of me. "Where are the stems?" she asked. "I ate them," I said with a shrug.

I did all of my favorite things. I talked to strangers just because I could. No need to be timid in English. I stopped in bookstores and thumbed through books for hours. I did everything that makes me happy. I took delight in the simplest of pleasures. I did everything I could to try to forget. To sit and reflect would feel like stepping into a void I might not come out of. I stayed busy—if I wasn't out in the London streets, I was laughing at a British comedy on the TV or reading a book. But try as I might, there was no forgetting that on July 12, everything would change. Nothing would ever be the same again.

6

Playboy for Breast Cancer and an Amputation

Coming back from London, I tried to focus on my upcoming surgery—do my due diligence, ask the right questions. I found an oncologist for a second opinion—I fell asleep during the two-hour wait in his waiting room. When he finally called me in, he glanced over the MRI images I'd brought and said, "What do you want me to say? You need a mastectomy. The charge is one hundred fifty euros." I paid him his fee for his five minutes of opinion.

I told some of my friends about my diagnosis, including my friend Liz, a fellow AUP alum, originally from Atlanta. "My mom is a breast cancer survivor. She'll be in town visiting if you want to talk to her," she offered. I was so grateful for the offer—I hadn't been able to talk to other breast cancer survivors, because I didn't really know any. The closest person to me with breast cancer had died years earlier, at age twenty-eight.

Not only was Liz's mother a breast cancer survivor, but she was also a doctor. A dermatologist, but, hey, beggars can't be choosers—it was more important to me that I would be speaking to a doctor without a language barrier. Someone who could help me understand.

I met with Liz's mom on a sunny afternoon at Le Pain Quotidien, of all places. We sat over coffee, and I listened intently as she told me about her journey with breast cancer. She never had a mastectomy, but it didn't matter—I was eager for any advice I could get. Being able to talk to someone who could understand was priceless. Thanks to the French medical custom of giving you your images after an exam, I had all of my paperwork with me. I took the MRI photos out of my bag, sliding them across the croissant-flaked table. "Here are my scans—what do you think about what they're suggesting?"

She held them up, examining them in the late afternoon sunlight. "I see what your doctors are saying—the lump is quite large," she said. She put them down and smiled sadly at me. "I think you should trust your doctors and do the mastectomy with immediate reconstruction."

It was a blow, but an expected one. With my second and third opinion in hand, as well as my own research, I needed to go ahead with the plan. I didn't see what else there was to do. The mastectomy was on.

◆ ◆ ◆

MY FAMILY ARRIVED. MY HAIR was freshly braided in two long boxer braids. My bag was packed. It was go time. If you read this in any other context, you'd think I was heading off to the hospital to give birth. Excitedly prepping for the new arrival in my life, nursery prepared to receive the bundle of joy. Except I wasn't going to gain anything. I was going to the hospital to lose something—my breast.

I woke up in a twin bed at 6 a.m., in an unfamiliar place. My family had rented an Airbnb so we could all be together for my recovery. There was so much lead-up to this day, these last moments. It was a whirlwind of activity and emotions. I wasn't afraid, though, only sad. I didn't know what to expect afterward; I had no point of reference. I didn't know anyone who had had a mastectomy before. The minute I tried googling anything, my nerves took over and I launched into an instant panic attack. I called friends and asked them to google for me—they vetted the information and passed it along.

I lay in the twin bed, staring up at the ceiling. It was unconceivable to me how much my life would change after today. I had had a blood test earlier in the week at the American Hospital. The nurse, engrossed in her clipboard, asked in stilted English about my breast cancer family history. "There's no family history of breast cancer," I said. She popped her head up over her clipboard to look at me. "Well, someone has to be the first," she said, snapping her clipboard closed.

Her words hit like a bullet to the chest. I sat in shock as she went forward with the blood test. Not only was my life changing, but my situation changed the lives of everyone in my family. It was me; I was the cancer. Nothing would ever be the same again.

I rose from bed and started getting dressed—a simple white and brown–patterned sundress that I picked because it was easy to get into and out of. As I stared down at my chest, looking at the traitors, a pang of resentment hit me.

I had always loved my breasts. I thought they were beautiful, perky, just the right size. It took a while for them to grow in, much to my disappointment, but at thirty-four years old, I felt they were exactly as they should be. I loved showing cleavage—there was a running joke about "the girls" with my NYC friends. But now as I looked down at the girls, there was one pretty breast on the right, and there was a Judas on my left. The Judas with the foreign body growing inside of it. The Judas with a biopsy scar right on top, forever ruining whatever cleavage I'd have after the surgery. It was hard to look at something I had once loved so much and now only felt disgust for.

I let the dress drop to my feet and went to the tiny window in the bedroom, which overlooked a courtyard. Using my phone, I tilted my head and snapped a photo. Then another. And another. I snapped until I had nearly twenty photos—forlorn, topless selfies of myself holding the two breasts I'd had and deeply loved for so many years. The pictures looked like the world's most depressing *Playboy* shoot—Hugh Hefner wouldn't be knocking on my door anytime soon. But I needed proof: evidence that I had existed in this way at one point in time. I wanted to see myself the way I was—even as I was mere hours away from it becoming a memory.

I pulled my dress back on.

◆ ◆ ◆

AFTER COMPLETING CHECK-IN, I SIGNED piles of paperwork in both English and French (one of the American Hospital perks). I signed an advance directive, saying if the surgery went wrong, I *did* want to be resuscitated. I signed financial paperwork, agreeing I'd be on the hook for the twenty-five-thousand-euro payment if my current insurance policy bailed on me.

And even on the day of surgery, there were more tests. Surgery day didn't mean that part was over. For hours I was poked, prodded, injected, and drawn on. They X-rayed me to find my lymph nodes—they would be removed to see if the cancer had spread there—and they marked the locations directly on me with a marker. I felt like a dry-erase board.

They asked several times, "Which breast is it?" to which I always responded louder than necessary, "The *left* one," with an exaggerated point to the offending boob. The only way this situation could be worse is if I woke up with my right breast gone, and I still have cancer. I suppose my tears could be dried by the euros won from the ensuing lawsuit, but I'd prefer to not have to go that route.

My entire family—Mom, Dad, and sister—came to the hospital. My sister's college roommate jokingly called us the "Swiss Family Robinson"—we went everywhere together. It was out of the question that my parents would come without my sister—or that only one of my parents would come. For something this serious, the Swiss Family Robinson had to be together.

My hospital room was a large corner unit. If it had been a hotel, I'd say I got upgraded. My favorite thing about the room wasn't the size or modernity, though, but the strong air conditioning blasting away the oppressive July heat. Every few minutes, nurses fussed around me, clucking their tongues and murmuring to themselves in French. They checked my IV and wristband, read clipboards, and strolled off. Some stopped to comment on the frigid temperature of the room—*"Il fait tellement froid"*—to which I just smiled. Allow me my small pleasures, please.

My parents went down to the gift shop, my father dropping an *InStyle* magazine I requested on my hospital bed. Glancing down at it, I saw the price was eighteen euros for a magazine that is normally six dollars in the US. I was shocked that my father, an accountant who could best be described as "frugal," would spend this amount of money on a magazine I'd read and toss. I could tell that my parents were worried—they were doing everything they could to stay calm and comfort me, including buying a nearly twenty-dollar magazine.

Dr. Toussaint, my oncology surgeon, walked into my room and paused to take in the scene. "The whole family is here, huh?" he asked, with a smirk. It was obvious it wasn't the norm to have the entire family with me—especially at thirty-four years of age. "They all wanted to come," I said, sheepishly. I was foolishly embarrassed to have so much support. He explained to my family how long the surgery would take and when they could expect to have me back in the room.

After hours of waiting and one family prayer, it was finally time. My family said their "see you laters" while hugging me, and my mother held on to my hand until the nurses rolled my bed away and our hands separated. I looked back at them, huddled together in the room, faces grim and sad, until they were out of my view. I was wheeled away from my room and pushed through the hallways of the hospital.

It was scary. Leaving my family—and seeing the concerned looks on their faces, especially knowing they were trying to put on a strong face for me—made me nervous. The feeling of not being in control of my body, the feeling I'd had since the diagnosis, was stronger than ever as I moved through the halls, boarding and riding elevators in my hospital bed. I was vulnerable—attached to so many wires and wearing a thin, half-opened hospital gown.

As I rolled through the halls, many other nurses and orderlies approached—some looking at my chart to see my native language and then asking in English, "Which breast is it?" Some didn't look at my chart and asked me in French. They asked many times in both languages, but the answer was always the same. Finally, an orderly leaned over me and smiled. "They're ready for you."

They rolled me into a blindingly white room—the kind of white that TV shows use to represent heaven. I squinted and raised a tethered hand to shield my eyes.

Doctors and nurses were everywhere, rushing around busily. The room was larger than my apartment—about the size of a small Parisian restaurant. Nurses filled tubes, pulled out bandages, and adjusted the operating table, while doctors checked and double-checked various items. Everything felt like a coordinated rhythm.

They spoke to each other over me in rapid-fire French—I was unable to understand a single word. It was jarring to see so many people bustling about. Were all these people really here for me? I was already scared, but the gravity of the situation sank in yet again—and the fear began to grow.

I'd only had one surgery before, and it had been under local anesthesia. Lying on the operating table in the clinic, I had listened to the doctor talk to the nurse about *Cold Mountain*, a new Nicole Kidman movie he had seen over the weekend with his wife. He told her the entire plot as he stitched up my ears after removing keloids. This was not the same. Not even close.

As they lifted me from the hospital bed to the operating table, I snapped back to reality. Everyone stared down at me with kind eyes. It was so much attention—too much attention, considering my butt was hanging out of a gown and I had marker scribbles all over my chest. I was (a bit late in the game) beginning to feel self-conscious.

Dr. Toussaint and Dr. Gauthier, the plastic surgeon who would do my reconstruction, showed up by my side. "Are you ready?" they asked, their eyes smiling as their mouths were covered with surgical masks. "No, but I guess we're doing it anyway, huh," I replied. Me being ready or not wouldn't change the outcome of the day. "Don't worry. It'll be okay," assured Dr. Toussaint.

The anesthesiologist came to my side and patted my hand. "It's important to think of something nice when you go under," he said. "It helps you come out of the anesthesia pleasantly and have good feelings. Think of a place you like to go to, or a place where you have fun."

Considering his words, I closed my eyes. My mind went to family vacations on the Delaware shore. Playing Scrabble at the dining table with my family, messily eating Maryland blue crabs at places with red-checkered paper tablecloths. Walking the boardwalk, on one side the Atlantic Ocean and on the other side a strip of stores selling everything from hermit crabs to beach towels. Watching kids ride the bumper cars, laughing at the surprise of the younger ones. Seagulls swooping aggressively for the fallen, well-seasoned Boardwalk Fries (who could blame them, they're delicious). Ice cream from Cold Stone Creamery on a hot day—or even better, a sundae from Dumser's Dairyland. Mini golf at locations scattered up and down Coastal Highway, some with dinosaurs, some with pirates, most with at least a waterfall or two. "Now count down backward from ten," the anesthesiologist said. And then it all went blank.

◆ ◆ ◆

MY EYES FLUTTERED OPEN—EVERYTHING LOOKED hazy and my mind was cloudy. I closed my eyes and opened them again. I was in a long, curtained room—a different room—one

I'd never seen before. I bent my fingers, wiggled my toes. I was attached to an IV bag that seemed to be different from the one I had had before. Even my hospital gown seemed different—newer. There was a clock across the room, but I had no idea what time it was. It seemed miles away. I didn't know how much time had passed: I could have been out five minutes or ten hours. Long, thick tubes spiraled out of the left side of my body, with plastic flasks at the end. Tucked under my hospital blanket, the flasks were filling with a mixture of blood and other bodily fluids. Drains. I cleared my throat—it hurt and felt dry.

"*Bonjour,*" I said, my voice coming out cracked and weakened. "*Bonjour,*" I repeated louder. A woman rolled over in a chair. "You're awake," she responded in English, stating the obvious and jotting notes on her clipboard. "*Oui,*" I responded groggily. "English? *Ou français ?*" she asked, her eyebrows knitted in concern. "*Oui, anglais*—yes, English," I responded. For unknown reasons, French came to me first upon waking from the surgery, so I understood her concern.

She wheeled over to her desk and walked back with a cordless phone. "It's the doctor," she explained, handing the phone to me. Dr. Toussaint's voice boomed across the line asking if I was okay. He said the surgery went well and he'd give me the details later. He said my throat hurt from the breathing tube they'd inserted during the surgery. I hung up feeling a bit unsettled—once again, I understood this surgery was a bigger deal than I'd realized. What else had happened while I was out?

After hanging up, I asked to call my family. I knew they

were worried, and I was excited to speak to them. She dialed the hospital room and my mother answered immediately. "You're out—how are you feeling?" I could tell my dad and sister were huddled close by in the background, trying to listen. "Yeah, I'm out—I'm okay," I said. Honestly, I could have been on an alien planet with three heads and I wouldn't have known. The anesthesia was still doing its thing, and I didn't know up from down.

We hung up and I immediately dozed off while waiting to be brought back to my family. The biggest part was done. Now we played the waiting game. We needed to see the tumor and lymph-node test results. This would decide if it was the beginning of my journey—needing chemo or radiation—or if it all ended here.

◆ ◆ ◆

I STAYED IN THE HOSPITAL for several days. I was glad to be there instead of recuperating at home. I didn't have to change the bloody plastic flasks tethered to my side, and I could enjoy the air conditioning. I was lucky, and I knew it: in the US, a mastectomy is an outpatient procedure for many women, emptying their drains in their bathroom sinks while being in so much pain they can barely move. My mother stayed by my side the first night, sleeping in a hospital chair.

In the hours following the surgery and the next day, I didn't feel much pain due to the anesthesia. When it finally began to wear off, the pain was blinding. I didn't want to use the morphine button they put in my bed—I always hated taking medicine. The nurses clucked their tongues at me. "If you don't use it and are in pain, your blood pressure goes up and it makes your recovery worse," they explained. I begrudgingly pushed the button, shooting the drug directly into my IV. I had my moments of confusion with the morphine—happy confusion, but saying things that didn't make sense. But at least I didn't have any pain.

The plastic surgeon had said that the reconstruction surgery would consist of lifting my pectoral muscle from the chest wall and putting the implant directly underneath—but it felt like they had rammed a watermelon into a piece of pita bread. A cantaloupe into a tortilla. A basketball into a manila folder. You get the idea. And with all the bruising, it looked like it too. It wasn't like in the US where implantation was done gradually with spacers—a process I heard is painful, but I'm not sure which process is worse.

At night in my hospital bed, the cacophony from the various medical machines I was attached to kept me awake; I blasted a mix of Sia and Hans Zimmer in my earbuds to drown it out. It didn't help that every thirty minutes a nurse would wake me up by checking my vitals.

In addition to the pain I was in and drugs I was on (both negatives for me, but you may feel differently), it sucked being in the hospital during this time of the year. Paris summers are magical. There is nothing like living in Paris during the months of May, June, and July. Paris gets up to sixteen hours of sunlight, the sun shining until almost 11 p.m.—and Parisians put that time to good use. The energy in the city puts even NYC summers to shame. And unfortunately for me, this summer was more magical than most.

Bastille Day, the July 14 celebration of the storming of the Bastille prison that marks the beginning of the French Revolution, was one of my favorite holidays. France goes all out for the holiday—it is essentially their Fourth of July. The day starts with a parade down the *Champs-Élysées*, complete with everything from army tanks to horses. A military band and choir perform the national anthem, "*La Marseillaise*," and one year even included a few Daft Punk hits. The parade ends with a fighter jet flyover in the French colors of blue, white, and red. There's even a televised battle reenactment—honestly, the strangest part of the whole day. Bastille Day ends with a fireworks show at the Eiffel Tower—a strong contender for one of the best pyrotechnics shows in the world. I watched every year with childlike awe.

This year, I wouldn't be at the foot of the Eiffel Tower on the *Champs de Mars* watching fireworks with a glass of champagne in hand. I wouldn't be watching the late-morning jet flyovers, leaving smoky streaks of blue, white, and red across the sky. On Bastille Day 2018, I was in the hospital. I still wanted to enjoy the day, so I asked the nurses if there was a place to watch the fireworks. That evening, I went to the rooftop in my hospital gown, attached to an IV, and viewed the display from there. My family joined me, but we weren't the only ones with that idea, as a few other gowned hospital patients in varying levels of health joined us. The rooftop view was amazing, but it didn't make up for how I would normally enjoy the holiday. It was still only two days after my surgery, however, and I had to make the best of it.

But Bastille Day wasn't the only thing I missed out on.

The World Cup was that summer—and France was one of the biggest stars of the tournament. From the start, I rooted for the French National team and faithfully watched every soccer match in bars with my friends, screaming my head off at the goals and cowering in anxiety during penalty kicks. I was all in. France was set to play Croatia in the final—the worst possible match to miss.

And I didn't plan on missing it.

I brought tiny French flags and face paint to wear in the hospital. On game day, I painted the French tricolor on my face and planted my flags on the sides of my hospital bed. The hospital staff found it hilarious—some even let me paint their faces. We chatted excitedly in "Franglais"—a mix of *français et anglais*. Many of the nurses popped their heads in to watch a few minutes of the match with me, yelling *"Allez les Bleus,"* the rallying cry of the French team. It was only three days after my surgery, and I had to make the best of it.

France won the World Cup and the French took to the streets, celebrating with music, dancing, honking horns, and the occasional car- or trash-can fire. Friends in the US, not knowing about my diagnosis and surgery, sent me a flurry of messages: "It must be wild to be in France right now! You're so lucky with everything going on," they said. "Yes!

It's a great time to be here. It's so exciting," I responded enthusiastically from my hospital bed, faking it.

Even my family was swept up in the magic. They arrived breathlessly the next day in my hospital room, regaling me with stories of people celebrating in the streets after the World Cup win—dancing on top of cars and hugging strangers. The city thrummed with electric energy. It was a big moment, it was *our* big moment—and after all the matches I watched, screaming my throat hoarse for *Les Bleus*, I missed the entire celebration.

Also, three days after my surgery, I had missed out on what I considered an opportunity of a lifetime. I missed seeing "Queen B." Beyoncé was in Paris for the On the Run II tour and the worst part? I had tickets. And they weren't just any tickets. They were *good* tickets. I'd only seen Beyoncé in concert before with Destiny's Child—a free mini show on the *Today* plaza. I wasn't a Beyhive member, but I knew she was a good performer. Being in France allowed me to get amazing seats without having to sell a kidney—I paid only eighty euros. Having such good tickets to the show, with seats close enough to count the moles on her face, for less than a hundred dollars—for me, it would have been a once-in-a-lifetime situation.

But instead of dancing and singing along to "Crazy in Love," I was in the hospital. A nice hospital, yes, but still a hospital.

After five days, I was discharged. My drains were removed—the bloodied flasks at my side finally taken away. It was an experience I don't wish on anyone. I screamed out for Jesus as the nurse pulled the long tubes out—and painfully felt every inch of it snaking out from the center of my chest. My scream could have awakened the dead in the morgue below.

I stepped out of the hospital, back in the same brown and white dress I had arrived in. My first time wearing real clothes in days. A folder full of aftercare instructions and prescriptions to be filled in my hand.

We went to the pharmacy down the road from our Airbnb when my father pulled me to the side, a stack of painkiller prescriptions I couldn't pronounce in my hand. "Sweetheart, don't worry about paying for your meds. I'll handle it," he said. I could tell he was worried about the cost—the list of medications was intimidating—and I had an around-the-clock schedule of painkillers and antibiotics to take. In the US, these same prescriptions could easily cost hundreds of dollars—there was no telling what the bill could be here.

At the register, we braced ourselves for an exorbitant price tag. "*Trente euros, s'il vous plaît,*" the pharmacist said, handing over my white paper bag of meds. Thirty euros. My father looked at me in shock and then back at the register. Yet another upside of French healthcare—the cost would have been far more than thirty dollars in the US, especially since the prescription included ketamine. My father paid, and we thanked the pharmacist. Dad wouldn't get over that shock for the rest of his time in France.

Despite my twenty-four-hour medication schedule, I planned to go back to work soon—I had asked for only two weeks of sick leave, the least possible amount. I needed to show my job that I was dedicated: worthy of being given a longer contract, worthy of being seen as someone to keep around. Because if I wasn't given a longer contract, who knows what could happen to my residency and health insurance, two things that held so much importance now.

Days later, I went back to the hospital to meet with Dr. Toussaint and discuss the test results. "Your lymph nodes showed no sign of cancer. The margins were tight but seem clear. No need to get chemo or radiation—you're fine," he said. Seated next to me, my parents rejoiced. "See what God did," my father said as we left the hospital. "God is good," my mother agreed. But if everything was all good, why did I still feel so empty? "Yep, it's great," I said, wiping away fallen tears. I couldn't explain the feeling—why I didn't feel as happy as my parents. Maybe it would take time for the news to settle in. Maybe my hormones were all over the place from the surgery. Either way, I was still on that elevator again. And it felt like this time, I'd reached the bottom.

7

You Don't Know What You Don't Know

Summer ticked along as I recovered. My parents watched the last leg of the *Tour de France* roll into Paris before returning to the States and leaving me to settle back into a routine.

The thing about cancer is that life doesn't pause for you when it arrives. Everything is still moving at breakneck speed while you're fighting for your life—or recovering from the fight of your life. Surgery was over and I was cancer-free, but so many people expected life to move on as before. And it was hard to explain that, yes, I am free from cancer but also, yes, I am tired and I am in constant pain. Pain that seemed like it would continue daily for the rest of my life.

Everything itched. Everywhere that a scalpel touched me had turned into grotesque lumps of scar tissue—keloids.

I knew I was prone to them—they were why my ears were operated on as a child and why I sadly never got the right-of-passage belly button piercing so many of my peers had. My keloids probably saved me from a lifetime of bad tattoo decisions too, so you have to look on the bright side.

My left arm tingled and burned. I was plagued with daggers of shooting pain—nerve damage from severing thousands of nerves when they amputated my breast and removed my lymph nodes.

I had to learn how to sleep again. A dedicated stomach sleeper, I couldn't take the pressure on my chest now from sleeping on my stomach. I felt like I was sleeping with a bomb strapped to my chest—my implant was firm, but I worried my weight could burst it. I googled late at night, feeling anxious in bed as I watched videos of trucks running over breast implants. Nothing to worry about, the videos said, as they dropped implants from the top of a building. Nothing will burst it.

I walked with a slight hunch on my left side. My muscles were taut—tight enough to snap. I wouldn't dare carry my purse on that side, and a backpack was completely out of the question. I couldn't lift my arm above my shoulder: even lifting it to my shoulder hurt. I held my arm in front of my chest when moving about the city. Parisians (and tourists) often bump your shoulders while jetting about the city without a simple "excuse me." A shoulder bump would leave me in pain for hours, so I moved slowly through the city, gingerly cradling my arm to protect myself.

In addition to the daily pain, there was also a feeling of

absence. I couldn't feel my breast anymore. It's like nothing existed there.

The pain wasn't only physical. I wasn't happy with the aesthetic results of my surgery. My reconstructed breast was smaller than my natural one and felt bolted onto my chest. It was firm and high. I avoided mirrors whenever getting dressed, not wanting to see the reminder of what I had gone through. I felt deformed, ashamed. My body betrayed me and these scars, this deformity, this monstrosity on my chest would always remind me of that.

I went for a follow-up appointment with Dr. Boucher. I took off my shirt and she examined my chest. "Wow, they're great. They did a wonderful job," she murmured. "Really?" I exclaimed, unable to hide my surprise. "Yes, I've seen a lot of them and this looks quite good," she said. I felt crushed. This was a good result—a great result? I was so disgusted by my chest, but apparently this was as good as it would get. Also: did she not remember my previous rack? Definite downgrade.

In front of others, I pretended it didn't bother me—a pattern I'd started to notice since the whole cancer journey began. I eagerly lifted my shirt to show the "French boob" to friends. I sent pics on WhatsApp to curious friends. Sadness, pain, and discomfort only make other people uncomfortable. I'd caused my loved ones enough pain with my diagnosis—I could put up a façade to make them happy. No need for all of us to be depressed over my boobs.

I found my escape in books. I read as much as humanly possible. I read in bed, I read on the Métro, I read while watching TV (weird, I know). I was always an avid reader but now I read with an intensity—a desperation. Reading was the only thing I could do where my mind wasn't hung up on cancer, fear, and pain. I lost myself in my books, from Jodi Picoult to Angie Thomas to Jon Krakauer. Only once I closed the book would the feelings rush back like a tide coming into shore.

I returned to work after the two weeks of sick leave that I allowed myself. I even trudged into work once during those two weeks due to an "important" brainstorming meeting that had appeared on my calendar from my boss. I wasn't typically invited to anything from the head of the department, so I chugged my meds and made the effort to go in (had to show myself as valuable, remember!), despite my family's disapproval. Turns out *everyone* was invited, so I was not at all special, and I almost passed out from the pain and exhaustion on my way back home, calling my family while sobbing in the streets, unable to take any more steps, asking them to get me and take me back to the Airbnb.

Commuting to work by Métro during rush hour was the worst. Line 9 was notoriously crowded, and the crush of people meant protecting myself was difficult. My best attempts still led to discomfort at best and pain at worst. I'd sit when a seat would become available, protecting myself from others' casual bumps.

One day a man stood over me, screaming in French that my seat should be given to someone else. No one knew what I was dealing with—to them I looked like a young, fit woman stealing a seat from the more deserving. In this case, he felt a woman with her five-year-old child was more deserving. He berated me over and over in French as everyone stared. Thankfully, I couldn't understand him completely, but I got the spirit of his tirade. Paris was not a hospitable environment for my recovery, but fortunately I could always go home. And I did.

I flew to the US in August, a month after my surgery, using vacation days to recover and soak up the love of family and friends for a few weeks. Yet another thing I was thankful to France for: generous vacation time (six weeks a year, to be exact). I could continue to recover in the comforts of home. No men screaming at me on public transport, no giving in to urges to go to the office to seem like a superhuman employee.

On the plane, I felt for my purse at my feet but couldn't reach it. I tried over and over, stretching my hand into the tiny space in front of my seat. It wasn't until the fifth try that I realized my tray table was down and I was repeatedly slamming my reconstructed breast into the table—using the tray table like a meat tenderizer—in my attempts. I still couldn't feel a thing. I'm sure my seatmate thought I was a masochist.

At home, it felt good to be taken care of again, not having to worry about lifting heavy things or cooking when I was tired. But it also meant I could get more resources—resources I would understand in my native language.

I made an appointment for a breast cancer bra shop in NYC. I'd been wearing a compression bra since the surgery, but I knew I needed new garments. I had been instructed to toss my underwire bras after surgery, so I didn't have much left to wear. I found numerous posts online about this particular shop and their wide variety of specialty bras. They understood breast cancer survivors. It would be my first foray into the survivorship world, a world I didn't quite feel like I belonged to.

After taking the train from DC to NYC, I made my way to the shop, dodging tourists and office workers in Midtown East. I rode a tiny elevator up to the boutique, located in an office building. It felt like I was going to the dentist more than a bra shop. After a few tentative raps on the door, I was greeted by a woman with a shock of wavy hair and bright red plastic glasses. The shop was small: no more than two rooms, one filled with racks and drawers of nude-colored undergarments. "Nude" that would never match my skin—another observation I had about the breast cancer survivor world.

"Come on in and wait a few minutes while I'm with the other women," she said. I stepped into the shop, taking it all in. I was the youngest and the only Black person in the room, a common observation since my diagnosis. Older white women, some with short hair and some with long, filled out forms and fingered the bras on display.

I hoped I would be in a place where a sense of belonging would kick in. *I'm with people who will understand my story, no matter how short it was.*

But instead, I felt like an imposter, taking up space in this shop meant for real survivors. I was just a woman who had had a mastectomy and then continued with life. I didn't feel like one of them.

"Okay, I'm ready for you." The woman with the red glasses stepped into my line of vision, a tape measure around her neck. "Let's go into the fitting room." She pulled back a curtain, and I entered and began to disrobe. As I took off my top, I began to explain my situation.

"I was diagnosed two months ago—in France, where I live," I said. "I had a single mastectomy on the left side last month, and I've only been wearing the compression bra." My story spilled out of me in a rush. She approached me with the tape measure, wrapping my body gingerly in the tape. She held a short pencil in her mouth and furrowed her brow in concentration. "So, I'm excited to get a new bra to wear; I don't have any others," I continued.

Red Glasses held the measuring tape on my side, lengthways. She wrapped me again in the tape, gently, the way a woman who has experience with survivors would do. "So, what about after surgery? Radiation? Hormone therapy?" she mumbled through the pencil dangling in her mouth. It was her first interruption to my blathering. "No, no radiation, no hormone therapy," I answered.

Red Glasses dropped the tape and stepped back, eyebrows raised. "You didn't do any radiation or hormone therapy?" "Um, no, they said I didn't need to do it," I replied. A curious look crossed Red Glasses' face—her mouth downturned and eyebrows raised. It was a look of both pity and confusion. "Humph," she muttered.

She wrote a few notes on her notepad, not looking back at me again. My face flushed—had I said something wrong? I didn't understand her reaction. My doctors told me I was fine—I had to trust them as I had nothing else to go on. No one else in my family had breast cancer, and if my doctors said I was fine, I was fine, right? My face was warm with embarrassment.

Red Glasses explained that the bra would be ready for pickup in a couple of weeks. I had walked into the shop excited and confident. I walked out of the shop insecure and panicked. I felt worse leaving than I did entering. Should I ask for more treatment? Were my doctors wrong? What did this woman know that I didn't know? I mumbled thanks to Red Glasses and took the paper—but I knew I wouldn't be back.

◆ ◆ ◆

IT WASN'T THE FIRST TIME that I realized you don't know what you don't know. And it applies to cancer in general, but specifically, the French healthcare journey.

Coming back to the office after my recovery in the US, my cancer was like a dirty little secret—I only told one person at work, for fear that I would lose my job. The domino effect could have devastating effects on my life. Losing my job meant losing the residency visa that was tied to my job, thus losing the only health insurance I had. The level of urgency that guided my actions pre-cancer to get this job ramped up even higher. I had one more reconstructive surgery ahead of me: I couldn't afford to lose my residency and health insurance.

Bills were piling up—all the medical tests and operations that were paid via credit cards were coming back on me hard with an astronomical interest rate. My take-home pay of three thousand euros a month barely kept me afloat with the credit card bills on top of the norm. I did get reimbursements for some of my medical expenses, but not for the full amount. Plus I was stretched so thin while waiting six weeks for the reimbursements that I had to rely on credit cards again for living expenses.

I had struggled earlier in the year while trying to find a job in Paris, and my savings had dwindled—now that I had a job it seemed unfair that I was still underwater. I didn't want to ask my parents for help: flying over for the surgery wasn't cheap, and they had paid for me to visit the US in August.

Back in Paris, I needed to find some way to relieve the financial pressure. I ended up selling my camera—the Canon DSLR I bought to help launch my freelance career in Paris. It added to the list of the many ways I felt like a failure, one of the many things that cancer stripped from me. Not only did I need to sell it to make money, but I also had problems filming with it due to my shoulder and back mobility issues from the surgery. It became an expensive paperweight that I couldn't afford to keep. Letting it go felt like the end of a dream.

I posted the camera for sale online, and a young guy with his own production company met me to purchase it. Turned out, his business partner was on leave because of his own extended battle with cancer. What was meant to be a brief ten-minute LeBonCoin purchase turned into an hour-long talk over coffee. I left the transaction feeling lighter—I'd unloaded both my camera and my trauma, plus pocketed a thousand euros to go toward my bills.

But that payday didn't mean the end of my financial

problems. I went to my *mairie*—the city hall for my neighborhood—and met with social workers, explaining slowly in French the details of my situation. The social worker, a young woman, listened to me intently and explained that she was, even as a French person, also confused as to why my reimbursements weren't the full amount. The French healthcare system is good but not exactly transparent when it comes to the finances of major health situations. The *mairie* mailed me a two-hundred-euro check to help me pay expenses. It was embarrassing—I had never had financial problems to this level before. I never had to ask anyone for help. I considered bankruptcy to get me out of the hole.

The thing about feeling like you've hit rock bottom after cancer is that no one wants to hear that. Any complaint you have, no matter how valid, is greeted with "But at least you're alive! You're healthy!" Well, so are you, but that doesn't stop me from listening to your life complaints. I couldn't complain about my financial stress—most people would respond, "Imagine how much it would be in the US." Which was true. I wasn't a hundred thousand dollars in debt from my medical treatment like so many people were in the US.

I didn't want to be seen as a victim—I didn't think I was—but I just wanted people to understand. Being in Europe doesn't make everything rainbows and butterflies. I wanted to vent without friends loudly proclaiming to me how my situation could have been much worse. I didn't need that perspective—I knew it. It was not a helpful tactic when you feel like you're drowning underneath the weight of it all.

At the height of my stress, with one more surgery planned for February, I made an appointment with the health insurance liaison at my job. I was assured she could help me with my new work insurance, which had finally kicked in, to get reimbursed for the upcoming surgery and tests I couldn't afford. The whole process was confusing, and no one offered to explain it to me. My phone calls and emails left me more confused than when I'd started and each medical appointment dwindled my account more and more. I was running out of credit cards to put everything on and still didn't have the money to pay them all back.

Finally, I'd get some help, the cavalry would come in. Salma, the health insurance liaison, sent brusque emails, but I figured that was her email style. I didn't have a good read on the communication styles at my job yet.

"So," I began, cradling a cup of coffee at the airy office café, "I was diagnosed with cancer, and I have lots of tests and surgeries to pay for. It's been a real strain on me, and I'm wondering what I can do to get the insurance to cover more of it." Salma stared back at me with obvious disinterest. Her eyes didn't become warm at the mention of cancer—she seemed more annoyed than anything.

"So, what do you want me to do about it?" she asked.

She blinked. I blinked.

"Well, I'm confused as to what is being covered. My doctors gave me the *affection long duree* status, which means I should have all of my tests and surgeries covered—what is happening?"

Talking to Salma was like talking to a brick wall.

Honestly, a brick wall would have had more give. "Well, you're going to an expensive hospital and doctors, so what do you expect? Why aren't you going to the public hospitals?" Her tone was accusatory and her voice boomed through the café—the cavalry she was not. "Because it's who my doctor recommended, and I didn't have my *Carte Vitale*—I didn't know there was a difference and I'm not fluent in French. No one told me any of these things," I stammered.

She sighed loudly. "Why aren't you negotiating with your doctors? I don't understand why you didn't negotiate the fee with them; that's why you're paying so much," she said. "Negotiate?!" I asked, my voice cracking. My lower lip trembled and tears began to spill, crying in anger. I hated that I was crying in front of this unsympathetic and brash woman—and also in the office coffee shop—but here I was, tears rolling down my face.

"I'm from the US. We don't negotiate with the doctors—we negotiate with the insurance. I didn't know any of this!" I shrieked. No need to worry about her causing a scene in the coffee shop, my hysteria had already turned a few heads.

How could I be expected to do things that I didn't know about and much less had never heard of? Negotiating with my doctors like my health was for sale at a bazaar? Gambling with my health for the lowest bidder? It's not like I was seeking treatment for a common cold. This was cancer.

Salma, full of a never-ending supply of sighs, didn't offer a napkin or anything for my tears. Only more sighs. I was certain that the only reason she wasn't rolling her eyes was because our meeting was in person. "Well, do that," she insisted.

I ended the meeting—there was no reason to continue to talk to someone who was annoyed by my presence, existence, and lack of knowledge of the French healthcare system. How she got a job like this, the world may never know.

• • •

ONCE I FELT STRONG ENOUGH that the mere sight of the words "breast cancer" wouldn't cause me to spiral, I sought out the counsel of online support groups. Typing in "breast cancer" in the Facebook search bar brought up tons of results. I joined the top three groups and waited for the supportive feelings to start.

I took my time before saying anything in the groups. I lurked, reading post after post of women lamenting their surgeries or, even worse, their chemo side effects. Women said matter-of-factly that they only had a year to live. Some women posted religious memes, to inspire everyone to continue the fight. Everyone seemed so strong, so determined. Scared, yes, but they exhibited the fortitude that I felt I was lacking. I was a fraud—I'd only had an amputation, so was I really a survivor? I didn't see what we had in common.

After weeks of lurking, I commented on one woman's post, asking for our cancer experiences. I wrote about my DCIS diagnosis and subsequent surgery, and how things are fine now—no more cancer. Almost immediately, there was a deluge of replies:

"What stage were you?"

"Were you ER+ or PR+?"

"What about your oncotype score?"

The responses flooded in and I wasn't ready. And it wasn't just that I wasn't ready, but I didn't know the answers. What is ER or PR? What is an oncotype? My stage? I was told I didn't have a stage. It was a precancer. Some didn't even consider it real.

The information overload overwhelmed me. My breathing deepened and my eyes welled up with tears. I didn't know any of this information and wasn't sure why I didn't. Everyone else seemed to have a strong handle on all their cancer facts and stats, and yet I was lost. I was used to feeling lost in France—it was par for the course for many expats—but to feel lost in my native language was worse. I was ignorant, and there was no worse shame than that. I slammed my laptop shut, angry at the Facebook group, angry at myself.

Maybe I had stuck my head in the sand. I was the common denominator here, so it must have been all my fault. I tried to stay afloat, to ask the right questions. I had asked for second and third opinions before surgery. Had I not done enough?

Going through cancer alone, in a foreign country, while working full-time meant mentally that I was swamped. I tried to keep all of my appointments straight, gather the paperwork needed, translate it all (medical paperwork can be difficult even in your native language), and excel at my job so I wouldn't lose my healthcare, all while trying to remain calm and not lose my mind.

No one who knew how everything worked—cancer, the

French healthcare system—was around to help me navigate it all. I didn't have a French boyfriend or husband that so many expat women had, who could come to appointments with me or advocate for me in French. How much did I miss? How many things had slipped through the cracks?

I reopened my laptop. I deleted my comment and clicked "leave group" on all the support groups. My ignorance shamed me. It was only three months since my surgery and four months since my diagnosis. Maybe I wasn't ready to confront what I'd gone through. I thought I had a handle on things, and I was ready to forge ahead, move on. But you don't know what you don't know.

◆ ◆ ◆

THROUGHOUT IT ALL, I WAS still dealing with apartment drama.

Things had improved after my first spot—my little parking space of an apartment in Saint-Germain-des-Pres. After only three months of living in the tiny studio, I moved to a larger, newer studio in the 8th arrondissement, close to the bustling Saint-Lazare train station. The studio was sunny and airy, with a top-floor balcony and large bathroom. The landlord was a photographer, and the apartment was well decorated with art from her travels and photos she'd snapped.

I loved that apartment.

I had finally found a true home. I was in my last year of grad school and hosted study groups and *apéros* and enjoyed cozy nights at home. There was still a sofa bed, but the owner provided high-quality furniture—these weren't odds and ends picked up from friends and family like so many other apartments. The bed was plush and comfortable, and my kitchen was clean and modern. I had my own oasis in Paris.

After my UNESCO internship for my master's program ended, I knew if I was going to stay in Paris, I needed a job and needed it *soon*. I couldn't survive on student loans forever and my thirteen-hundred-euros-a-month rent was shrinking my savings quicker than expected. So after one and a half years in the dream apartment, I decided I needed to move if I was going to make The Paris Plan sustainable for a few more years.

I went back to my university's housing database, browsing the available apartments. An apartment in the 16th arrondissement caught my eye—twelve hundred euros a month for a one-bedroom. Sure, the 16th was boring and full of elderly, rich, snobby French people, but I needed cheaper rent. Sacrifices had to be made.

I arrived at an iron-gated Haussmannian building on a quiet, tree-lined street. A cobblestone path led to oversized mahogany doors with gold details. It was an old-money place—the type of place I'd never lived in before.

I met the landlord, an elderly Parisian man with excellent English, and walked through the massive gold-detailed door into the well-kept courtyard and a gorgeous eight-story building stood before me. I was walking toward the iron-gated door when the man cried out, "Oh no, it's not that building. It's this building." I turned my head toward him—he gestured to a tiny, dilapidated doorway. "It's the service entrance," he said with a smile.

Feeling like a second-class citizen, I followed him, ducking into the doorway and walking past the trash bins. We rode the rickety elevator up to the dark and dank sixth floor. "You have your own toilet," he boasted. "Most of the tenants on this floor share the toilet," he said, pointing to a tiny doorway in the hall. The sixth floor, unlike the main building, had about twelve apartments—mostly studios with students or families piled in. The main building had only one or two grandiose apartments on each floor.

"The apartment was redone by an architect," he said, showing me around the cramped loft studio. "I normally rent it to two people at a time for twelve hundred euros, as it's a two-bedroom, but I can give you a deal." My eyes bugged at that piece of information—how could two people share this space? The apartment wasn't a true two-bedroom—it wasn't really a one-bedroom, in my opinion.

Steep stairs in the apartment led to a lofted area with a bed directly beside the stairs, without a safety wall, only a railing. God forbid I have a violent nightmare—which I was known to have—or I could find myself at the bottom of the steps with a broken neck. When sleeping on the bed, the ceiling was just two feet from your face. There were two alcoves to the side of the bed, where you had to crawl to gain access. One of those was considered the second bedroom. Tiny square windows in the apartment looked directly up to the sky, giving the feeling of being locked up in a tower.

But I needed cheaper rent to keep The Paris Plan going. The landlord invited me to his apartment (which I accessed via the servants' stairwell), and we sat in his grand salon and negotiated rent. His salon was twice the size of my entire apartment.

In the end, I rented the place for nine hundred euros a month—cash payment only. I made seven hundred and fifty euros a month at my internship at the communications agency, so I didn't have to dip as hard into my student loans as I did for my current apartment.

And for a while, it worked. I didn't love being a second-class citizen—using the creepy entrance and lurking about the building on the servants' stairwells—but it wouldn't be forever. My commute to work was a five-minute walk across the street—a benefit for some, but a disadvantage for me. It was impossible to shake the feeling of being at work all the time. As my work environment turned more and more toxic, the short commute depressed me.

After my mastectomy, the apartment became more of a problem for me. I couldn't crawl up the stairs after my surgery—I started to sleep on the sofa bed. With my back seizing in pain from the surgery, I was too afraid that I'd fall out of the bed and down the stairs—and ultimately to my death. I began the hunt for a new apartment: a place I could stay in for years and really make my own.

❖ ❖ ❖

AT FIRST I BELIEVED I'D found it: the place where I could happily spend a few years in Paris before buying an apartment to call my own. Tucked away on a side street near the *Sacré-Cœur* Cathedral, the studio was in a new arrondissement for me, the 18th. I was excited to live in the famed Montmartre neighborhood, climbing the hills and getting lost in the little charming streets.

The owner, a young Frenchwoman, had bought the Parisian studio before her career moved her to America. The apartment had good vibes. It was small—slightly larger than my parking-space apartment on *Rue Princesse*—but it had been renovated for maximum space.

The one-room apartment had an open floor plan, and the sleeping space—with an actual bed—was partitioned from the living room area with a Crittall wall. The furniture and decorations were trendy and funky: a yellow couch, and an extendible wooden dining table for guests.

I toured the apartment with the owner's mother, starry-eyed. I was smitten. The apartment was cozy and cute. "I'm looking for a place I can feel good in," I said, perched on the edge of the yellow couch. After two years in Paris and multiple apartment visits, I knew Parisian landlords appreciated getting to know the prospective tenant's mindset and personality. I needed to sell myself.

"I've been through a rough time with my health recently, and I'm looking for a place with good vibes to aid my recovery—and I think I've found it," I added with a smile.

"There's a medical student living here now, but she's leaving soon to go back to Greece. You can move in a few days after she leaves," she said.

"I'd like to move in as soon as possible—can I move in the day after she leaves?" I asked.

The relationship with my landlord in the 16th had degraded. A massive leak had sprouted, but he told me it was my imagination (I quickly learned that I needed to document everything). He also frequently overstepped my boundaries. Despite his desire to be a grandfatherly figure to me, I was not his biggest fan. I particularly did not enjoy having to meet him for coffee each month in his apartment to hand him the rent in cash—a standing meeting that always led to him asking too much about my personal business. I missed the process in the US of renting directly from a company. I shouldn't have to make small talk about my life each time I paid rent.

"Sure, you can move in the day after—there won't be time for a professional cleaning to be done, but we can get the tenant to do a cleaning before she leaves."

So it was settled. I cheerily packed up my apartment to abandon my abode in the 16th arrondissement and start a new life in the 18th.

⁕ ⁕ ⁕

THIS MOVE WASN'T AS SIMPLE as the past two apartment moves—with each apartment, I had accumulated more belongings. Not to mention I often took advantage of my friends' giveaways when they left Paris: everything from blow dryers and flat irons to books I had yet to read. I spent the day lugging suitcases on multiple Uber rides across town—a task made more difficult by the never-ending *Gilet Jaunes* (Yellow Vests) protests—before finally collapsing onto the bed in my new apartment. It was exhausting, but I was happy to be in my new home. I fell asleep fast and hard.

Turns out, a good night's sleep wasn't meant to be. A banging noise jolted me out of my sleep—one bang, then several more bangs. I sat up straight in bed, removing my earplugs. The banging continued, my heart clanging in my chest nearly as loudly. My stomach flipping, from the bed I looked to the front door for the intruder—maybe this neighborhood wasn't that nice after all—but the door was still locked shut.

Suddenly, a mouse bolted from behind the couch, leaping onto the seat and running to the kitchen cabinets, squeezing itself out of sight. He had been rustling in the bag behind the sofa—a bag filled with the wooden slats for the extendable dining table—causing the banging noises.

I shivered, unable to speak, unable to make a sound. I closed my eyes and shook my head. Did I really just see that? Taking deep breaths, I was trying to calm myself down when another mouse darted out from under the very bed I sat on, scurrying to the kitchen cabinets. Oh hell, yes—I did see that.

Hyperventilating and shaking, I was frozen in fear. One mouse can happen—I had a mouse before in my Harlem apartment—but two mice? You officially have a problem. A mouse problem in an apartment the size of a one-car garage.

I called my mother immediately—it was only 8 p.m. there—crying into the phone. "I don't know what to do! There's mice in my new apartment; they're running all around," I sobbed. She was sympathetic but grossed out—and I was too terrified to sleep a wink that night.

It was reminiscent of when I moved to NYC, crying on the phone to my parents about that first apartment—infested with roaches and mold and frequently lacking hot water. My neighbors fought so violently that I couldn't keep a mirror or picture on our shared wall—that is, when they weren't in the hallway smoking weed. "You wanted to move to New York, this is what it is," my parents responded to my sobbing rants. Was Paris the same? Was this the type of living accommodations that I'd sentenced myself to?

There was nothing left to do but sit on my bed, with every single light blazing, waiting for sunrise. I stood sentinel all night long, blasting music as loud as I could at that time of night, trying to scare off any additional visitors. The night seemed endless as I waited for the 8 a.m. October sunrise. I could handle this; I'd dealt with worse.

The next morning, I immediately called the landlord's mother, who rushed over with an exterminator. I went to the hardware store, buying foam and steel wool. The exterminator would likely just put down traps—I also wanted to seal the holes to prevent my place from turning into a Mickey Mouse graveyard. There was no way I'd be able to empty traps myself anyway. I knew my limits.

I hired a handyman to work alongside the exterminator. I watched, head tilted over his shoulder, as the exterminator laid traps in the kitchen, which took up one wall of the open-floor-plan studio.

"What about the front door? There's a weird patch in

the corner of the front door," I asked, pointing to a circular area at the bottom that appeared to be papier-mâchéd together. *"Non, non, c'est définitivement la cuisine,"* he said, assuring me the kitchen was the problem. I was skeptical. The handyman dutifully followed behind his traps, stuffing steel wool into the holes in the kitchen area.

"I'm so sorry for this, but it should be fine now," the landlord's mother said. Either way, I was going to stay at Lyneka's for the night. I was exhausted and my nerves were shot. I jumped at every creak, every shuffling noise, every scratch. Sleeping in the apartment that night would be impossible.

The next afternoon, after a full night of sleep at Lyneka's, I returned to the apartment after work with Chelsea, my work friend. "Once in Canada, we lived in an old farmhouse and it had mice in the walls," she said. "We would hear them scratching around at night. So I'm not too afraid of all of that, I've been there before."

In the orange afternoon light, we tiptoed inside the apartment like robbers, keeping an eye out for signs of Mickey and friends. I needed to grab a few items of clothing for my next overnight stay—I still wasn't ready to return to the apartment for good.

As I was throwing clothes into a suitcase, a scratching sound in the apartment stopped us in our tracks. "It's from over there," I whispered, pointing at the kitchen cabinets. Chelsea's eyes widened as the scratching continued, louder and louder. So much for not being afraid—apparently the Canadian mice had nothing on French mice. And so much for my brilliant two-step extermination plan.

We hastened our pace, not wanting to see our scratching friend make his debut in the apartment.

The whole situation was depressing: I had gone from a bad situation to a worse one, which felt like the story of my life those days.

My stress levels, already high from health concerns, were skyrocketing. I was jumpy and anxious, not to mention depressed. Every day I felt on edge—like I was on the verge of a heart attack. When I had rodent issues in NYC, it was easily fixed: some poison here and there, sealing the holes, and you're fine. But much like their human counterparts, apparently Parisian mice were intent on living the good life—and doing so in my apartment. I was someone who always had a plan, but I didn't know how to fix this situation.

The next day, I ventured back into the apartment. I was going to Greece—my friend Nicola had invited me to tag along on her work trip for free—and I needed to get my luggage. The apartment immediately felt different when I stepped inside. It sounded different as well—a high-pitched squeal and rattling came from the corner of the studio. My diminutive non-rent-paying roommates were back. Tension and anxiety came bubbling to the surface—my heart was thudding out of my chest and I started to hyperventilate. I began to cry—silently at first, then sobbing. I ran out of the apartment, into the narrow hallway.

A woman, on her way out of the building, stopped on the stairwell upon seeing me. *"Qu'est-ce qui se passe?"*

"Il y a une souris!" I screamed, telling her there was a mouse. She looked at me with raised eyebrows, a puzzled

look on her face. *"Une souris!"* I said again, desperate for her to understand me. I know my French isn't the best, but I hated her in that moment for not picking up context clues. What else could I actually be saying?

The door next to my apartment opened, and a young blonde woman poked her head out. At this point, I'm the hysterical American dramatically sobbing in the hallway. If I planned to not make a scene, I failed one hundred percent. I was too distraught to care.

"Qu'est-ce qui se passe?" the woman asked me.

"Une souris," I wailed, too stressed to move beyond that one phrase.

"English?" she asked, detecting either my accent or my bad French or both.

"Yes! Yes! There's a mouse in my apartment! I just came home and he's in there and I don't know what to do."

The neighbor, more competent than me, charged into the apartment looking for the intruder. The rattling in the corner made it evident: a mouse was trapped in the oversized decorative planter, doing circles like a NASCAR driver. He must have climbed in but the sides were too slick for him to be able to climb out.

"Oh! He's cute," she said, peering into the planter. I stood in the doorway, still sniffling but trying to pull it together. I gave a fake chuckle at her response, hiding my disgust. Ma'am, please. There's nothing cute about a mouse.

"I'll take it to the window and let him outside," she said, lifting the heavy planter. I opened the window and she laid the planter down on the second-floor windowsill for him to run out—but I guess he had other ideas. "Oh no, he jumped! Oh no," she lamented. So much for saving his life—now I had a mouse suicide on my conscience.

I thanked my distraught neighbor and quickly gathered my belongings and left. No way could I stay in this apartment. But I wasn't looking forward to the battle that would ensue to get out of my lease.

Not only did the mouse situation continue to get worse, but the apartment was uninhabitable. The mice tore a hole in the front door, the same hole in the door I asked the exterminator about. They were desperate to get into my apartment—by any means necessary. I imagined them lining up like miniature medieval armies, storming my front door and kitchen cabinets. I ended up not having to go to battle: thankfully, the landlord offered to let me out of the lease and I accepted quickly.

I had hastily moved out of my last place in the 16th. In fact, I left that apartment so quickly that I still had a few weeks left on the lease. Under the cover of night, I started moving back into the apartment, hoping my landlord wouldn't see. One night, while I was loading suitcases onto the tiny elevator, he caught me red-handed. "Do we need to talk?" he asked, a smirk on his face. "We do," I said, bowing my head. I hated to give him this small pleasure, but I was out of options.

He let me move back into the apartment until the end of the year, then he'd want to have new tenants. The hunt for a new home began again.

8

Getting Even: A Tale of Two Titties (They Both Look Good!)

I accepted that I had cancer. I accepted my mastectomy. But what really concerned me was Tinder.

You read that right—yes, Tinder.

Let's back up a little bit. Dating in France was far more difficult than I had imagined, which is saying a lot, coming from the New York City dating world. When Rihanna sang, "We found love in a hopeless place," I had always assumed she meant NYC. The insane dating stories I had in NYC could be a whole separate book. But I'm in France—it should be different, right? Where is Pierre, whom I'd meet in my neighborhood *fromagerie*, reaching for the same melt-in-your-mouth *beurre salé*, locking eyes and forever changing the trajectory of our lives?

What about Armand, who would charm me at the *boulangerie* while waiting in line for a crusty but delicious baguette (*une tradition, bien sûr*)? Was it possible that I was fooled by the countless American-in-Paris books/movies/TV shows? Spoiler alert: I'd been fooled.

That's not to say that dating in Paris is completely abysmal. Pre-cancer, I went on dates with many wonderful men—some who wined and dined, some who surprised me at the end of an otherwise romantic night by splitting the bill ("I don't want to offend your feminism by offering to pay the bill"), and some who strolled the Parisian streets with me, discussing everything from culture to philosophy until 5 a.m., when the mouth-watering smell of *boulangeries* starting their morning bread routines greeted us.

There was the handsome finance man who took me to *Caveau de la Huchette*, the jazz club featured in *La La Land*, where we danced the night away in the cramped, sweaty basement, surrounded by swing dancers.

There was the beautiful elementary school teacher with a kind heart and piercing eyes, whose gaze made me feel like I was the only woman in the room.

Not to mention the dynamic communications professional who cooked me a delicious home-cooked meal in his cramped Parisian kitchen, equipped solely with a toaster oven—one of the best meals I'd had in Paris.

And then there was the pharmacist, a kind, older gentleman, who when I told him I preferred to be friends, responded, "To offer friendship to someone who wants love is to give bread to someone who is thirsty." I'd certainly never received such a poetic response to a rejection before.

Most of the men were bilingual—or if not, they were

intrigued by the idea of an American woman and loved the opportunity to improve their English. Even if I tried to have the date in French, they would insist we continue in English. So much for learning a new language via love.

My dating life was on a different level in Paris than in NYC, where I kept running into the same Peter Pan types (men who never want to grow up). But there were also differences that I could do without.

I went on dates frequently, but I rarely met anyone I wanted to see long-term. Despite yearning for partnership, I wasn't finding it—and I believed having the cancer baggage would make things worse.

There are many ways to describe the mix of tissue and fat hanging from a chest, "breast" being the most obvious. Tits, boobs, jugs, rack (but only if you have two!). And that's just off the top of my head. If you go to Urban Dictionary (reader beware, but I guess if you made it this far, you'll be okay), you'll find many more colorful expressions like honkers, hooters, knockers (I particularly like this one), melons, tatas, bust, and bosom.

But it all boiled down to this: how can I be titless on a dating app? If it's already hard out there for a woman who is darker than a paper bag (colorism is real and worldwide), over thirty, and not built like Megan Thee Stallion—how much harder is it for a woman with all of the above, but minus a real boob?

It's another thing that you're not "allowed" to worry about. Whenever I voiced my concern to a friend, whether venting or wanting support, I was told to "be happy you're alive" and that "the right one won't care." That's all fine and good, but is that really the case? I hoped it was, so during my mastectomy recovery, I fired up the app, timidly swiping a few minutes each day, giving my thumb the Tinder workout.

But before that—there was André.

I met André a few months before my initial diagnosis. His Tinder profile piqued my curiosity. He had various laughing and travel photos—he appeared to enjoy life and looked fun to be around. Our first date confirmed it: he was a well-traveled, open-minded, intelligent Frenchman who had a kindness that I didn't often encounter in the world of online dating.

André and I had a few dates, and I enjoyed his company but wasn't quite sure if I wanted to become exclusive. In the end, I wasn't given much of a choice in the matter. After a third dinner date at a hidden-jewel Asian restaurant, André walked me to the Métro, where we'd both get on our respective lines home. We swiped our Métro cards, going through the turnstiles. He turned to me, his eyes darting between the floor and my face. "So, what are we doing here? What's going on with us?" he asked as Parisians bustled all around us in the crowded station.

Unaccustomed to direct communication in the early stages of dating, I was flustered. And this was such bad timing. The Métro cars barreled down the tunnels as I moved side to side to avoid colliding with Parisians rushing to catch the train. The brakes screeched loudly as they pulled into the station.

The pungent urine smell of the Métro made me gag. My eyes darted around, wondering 1) Is this really happening? and 2) Is anyone else seeing this? "You're a nice guy. I like spending time with you," I stammered. "You're so nice," I repeated. I couldn't read his expression, but personally, I was mortified to have such an intimate convo on the smelly *quai* of the Métro. We said an awkward goodbye and I scrambled off to catch my train. I didn't hear from him again after that—and once I received my diagnosis four months later, I became too busy to care.

♦ ♦ ♦

I DESPERATELY WANTED TO FEEL normal again after my mastectomy, including dating again. I wanted to create as much emotional and mental distance as possible from my cancer journey—one I hoped was over. I wanted to hit the ground running. I reached out to André—I never fully understood why we fell out of contact in the first place.

I knew I could feel safe with him, which was above all what I needed. The cancer diagnosis rocked my world, and although things would never be the same, perhaps I could achieve some level of normalcy through this relationship. And for a while, it worked. The ever-agreeable André responded to my text and accepted my invitation to drinks. From that moment, it was on.

We saw each other several times a week, exploring Paris together—often with his Nikon camera in hand, snapping pics of the lesser-known parts of the city and sometimes of me. We went to art galleries and museums, movie theaters, and *apéro* parties with his diverse and gregarious group of friends. He was kind and gentle about my post-cancer appearance, telling me that it didn't matter to him.

But underneath it all, I still felt like a fraud. Breast cancer had a profound effect on my confidence and body image—my entire way of viewing the world and myself. We presented like a normal couple, but inside, I was ashamed of my cancer journey and the physical and emotional scars it left on me. Shouldn't I just suck it up and be happy that at least someone wants me?

◆ ◆ ◆

VALENTINE'S DAY WAS APPROACHING AND, for once, I was excited. I had plans—not with André, but with my plastic surgeon. It was time for my second reconstructive surgery. The best part of the surgery was that my stomach fat—fat I'd enjoyed putting on for this purpose—would be injected into the French boob for a softer and more aesthetically pleasing breast. The procedure, lipofilling, was a common next step after immediate breast reconstruction. Call me shallow, but I was excited. Perhaps after this surgery, I wouldn't avoid mirrors anymore or avoid seeing my body when out of the shower. And even better—it would be my last surgery. No more scalpels after this.

I still had follow-up appointments with the oncology surgeon, Dr. Toussaint, who was happy with the mastectomy results. He knew about my scheduled Valentine's Day plastic surgery with Dr. Gauthier and gave me a call. He explained to me that since my margins were so narrow, perhaps Dr. Gauthier could take a bit more breast tissue during this surgery. "Just to be on the safe side," he reassured me.

I was confused. To me, a mastectomy means there is no more breast tissue to take—it's all gone. Either way, I didn't think much more of it. Dr. Gauthier, with his new directive from my oncology surgeon, wouldn't be able to do the lipofilling, but he said he could swap out my current implant for a bigger one—so the surgery wouldn't be a complete waste aesthetically. I was disappointed that it meant it wouldn't be my last surgery—I'd still need the lipofilling done later—but it was a good compromise.

I wouldn't be spending Valentine's Day with André, but he seemed to understand. We'd been dating for about four months, so, in a way, it saved us from any potentially awkward first Valentine's Day plans. I was laser focused on getting this surgery done and out of the way—and finding out whether I still had cancer and would possibly need radiation or worse. This second surgery was crucial to my cancer journey. I relayed all this info to André and he appeared to understand, bobbing his head while listening to me. This surgery would be a moment of truth.

My mother flew to Paris—her first solo flight, at the age of seventy-one—to accompany me to the surgery and help me in my recovery. Preparing for the operation, I figured nothing could be worse than the pain of my mastectomy. I was ready to get it over with and be one step closer to being done with the whole ordeal. I checked into the clinic for my three-day stay. This time I wouldn't be in the upscale confines of the American Hospital, a choice made to help reduce out-of-pocket costs.

I wasn't well prepared for the surgery—it was hard for me to focus on many things these days. We waited in the clinic room, my home for the next three days. It was sparse but clean, and comfortable enough. They'd promised to wheel in a cot for my mother in the evening. She was a strict believer in staying the night with me after a procedure. I couldn't have kept her away if I tried.

A young orderly came in, an angel dressed in all white. Tall, chocolate, and young, about twenty-five years old or so—with a crisp fade and warm smile. Who knew Idris Elba was working in healthcare—certainly not me because I was *not* ready. "*Vous-êtes prêt?*" he asked. One thing I noticed about my time navigating the French healthcare system was that it could double for a model casting call. These people are beautiful. I'd never seen a parade of such attractive people working in hospitals until my mastectomy. Each nurse or orderly that came in was better-looking than the last. Again, am I shallow? Yes. Was it a good distraction from my problems? Also, yes.

This small Catholic clinic was no different. And it wasn't just my observation. My mother commented upon arrival, "There are so many attractive nurses here." The one difference was that this gynecological clinic employed mostly male nurses. Not that I was complaining.

"*Oui, je suis prêt,*" I replied to Nurse Idris Elba.

He lifted my arms, taking a peek at my armpits, and

lowered them with a cringe. *"Vous n'avez pas rasé?"* he asked. Confused, I turned to my mom—for unknown reasons since she does not speak French. *"Raser?"* I asked. No one told me I needed to shave my armpits before the surgery. I had so many scars and entry points that it didn't occur to me they would do the surgery via the long, thick scar in my armpit. *"Pas de problème,"* he said. He left the room, and I explained the situation to my mom.

Ten minutes later, Nurse Elba came back into the room, brandishing a disposable razor. He held up the razor triumphantly, with a shy smile. And much to my horror, this beautiful man proceeded to shave my armpits. Humiliated, I attempted to stop him, explaining in my broken French that I could do it myself. But it didn't matter—the most beautiful man I'd seen in a long time ended up sitting with his face in my armpit, slowly shaving with precision.

After everything I'd been through, I thought it was impossible for me to feel shame anymore. We sat there with both our cheeks flushed in embarrassment, avoiding each other's eyes, although we were just inches apart. This was not my preferred manner of closeness. *"C'est fini,"* he said with a smile, proud of his work.

They wheeled me down the hallway to the operating theater, a much smaller space than my previous one. I wasn't awed by the equipment or the bustling atmosphere. Everything was gray and shiny, not the gleaming white of the American Hospital. It didn't matter. I was one step closer to putting the whole ordeal behind me. I closed my eyes and counted backward from ten.

❖ ❖ ❖

I WOKE UP SORE AND confused in the hospital to reports of a successful surgery, my mother and my friend Isabelle by my side. The operation required a two-night hospital stay, but I was allowed visitors. My friends Beth, Catherine, and Liz came by with flowers, regaling me with funny stories to keep my spirits up. It felt like a high school sleepover, except in a hospital. Isabelle checked in on my mother and me often, making sure we had all we needed for my recovery. But who was absent? André. Yes, he texted me to ask how the surgery went, which I appreciated. But out of all of my hospital visitors, he wasn't one of them. Why?

He was throwing a party. While I was in the hospital, he was "unavailable" for two nights because he was throwing himself a birthday party. While I was laid up in bed, in pain, he was living it up with wine, charcuterie, and the aforementioned gregarious group of friends.

It was baffling and disappointing to me that someone who had shown himself to be sensitive and thoughtful was too busy having an *apéro* to even stop by for a couple of hours. It made me wonder if having a relationship was even worth it if I would still be going through the tough parts of life alone. He reached out the next day, before my release from the hospital.

"You're still at the hospital? Do you want me to visit this afternoon?"

"You can go party again, since that's what you like," I replied.

Things between us were never the same—it was the beginning of the end.

I gave myself another two weeks to recover from this surgery. Thankfully, there wasn't much to recover from—this surgery was much easier on my body than the mastectomy. After a few days of bed rest, I was up and about, receiving visitors and showing my mother around Paris. We went to a jazz concert where she did her first *bise*—the two-cheek-kiss Parisian greeting. Unfortunately, she didn't know a *bise* starts on the right cheek first and ended up kissing a friend of mine, a young jazz musician, square on the lips.

We spent our weekdays walking my neighborhood and our weeknights bingeing *This Is Us*. On Saturdays, we stayed in as the *Gilet Jaunes* held their never-ending protests all over France, setting fires to my neighborhood trash bins and dodging tear gas from the riot police.

We established a routine. We enjoyed ourselves—and I enjoyed her. She even started learning French via Duolingo: I often heard the app's chipper *ding* while in the clinic, my mom keeping her streak going and completing her lesson for the day. I enjoyed her company so much that I refused to book her return ticket to Maryland. It felt good to be taken care of and be with family. It was a morale booster, and I'm sure it contributed to my fast recovery.

But we didn't have the results of the biopsy yet.

My mother agreed to stay until my follow-up appointment, where I'd receive the biopsy findings. We went to see Dr. Gauthier in his office in the 14th arrondissement, not far from the Pantheon. Like with most of my breast cancer appointments, where I was often the youngest one in the waiting room and sometimes the only one with hair, his waiting room was no different.

But in this room, everywhere you looked, there was artwork portraying breasts—large, small, uneven, of all colors. It was the type of artwork where you couldn't immediately tell they were breasts unless you'd studied it for a while—which I often did during the up to one hour of wait time. There were breast sculptures, breast paintings, and breast photographs. White breasts, black breasts, pink breasts. Big breasts, small breasts, flower breasts. There's no way you could find yourself in the wrong office—his specialty was all over the walls.

I sat across from Dr. Gauthier's massive desk, scattered with handwritten notes, with a sculpture of breasts on the corner. Naturally. "The biopsy showed the margins weren't clear. The tissue we removed was cancerous," he said.

My mouth gaped open and my body went stiff. The world felt like it was shifting under my feet. I was thrown back to where I started in Dr. Boucher's office eight months earlier—it felt like a second diagnosis. I was stunned. Stunned and outraged. "So I still had cancer all this time?" I asked. "Yes, but we removed it and you're fine now," he said. I didn't expect this—it was shocking enough to be diagnosed with cancer the first time. But I had been given an all clear—told to go off into the sunset and enjoy life—when all along I still had cancer.

"Make an appointment with Dr. Toussaint to discuss, but I've spoken with him and it's okay. Now let me go take a look," he said, gesturing to his exam room behind me. Nothing made sense anymore. My health was still finding ways to shock me, even when I thought everything was okay. It was infuriating—and it was scary. And the worst part was that no explanation was given. No one sat me down to explain how this could have been missed. It was handwaved away as one of those things that could just "happen."

How could I trust anything? Could I trust my doctors? The sinking feeling in the pit of my stomach that opened in the bra shop in NYC was there again and filled with doubt. Should I have gone to the US for treatment? This news broke my trust in the French healthcare system. And it also broke my trust in myself.

I'd still had cancer from July to February and I never felt anything, never felt any sickness, never even doubted the doctors—so now I felt that I couldn't trust myself anymore. My judgment and my intuition were skewed. I was on a rollercoaster—back on the elevator—and I desperately wanted to get off.

♦ ♦ ♦

A FEW WEEKS LATER, ON a crisp spring day, I met André for a stroll along Canal Saint-Martin. After the shocking news that I'd still had cancer all along, I was reeling. Doubt and fear fought for first place in my mind on a daily basis. I couldn't focus on anything, and my grief and anxiety were overwhelming. I no longer had the mental and emotional bandwidth to be in a relationship, to be responsible for someone else's feelings. Everything within me needed to be poured back into myself.

I told André how I felt, speaking softly at first, then giving way to choked sobs on a bench by the canal. It was over between us. I didn't sob for the relationship but for myself. The pathology results rocked my world so violently that I didn't know whether I was coming or going.

"I didn't know what to say or what to do," he said.

"There's no manual on how to help your girlfriend through cancer," I replied.

While he was a special person, I realized I was forcing myself into the relationship just to prove I was okay. "I came through this unscathed, so I can have a boyfriend now. Everything is fine. It's all fine." When in actuality, I hadn't begun to process everything I went through. Not only was it unfair to him, but it was unfair to me as well. It was time to take another break from dating.

◆ ◆ ◆

LIFE, FORTUNATELY OR UNFORTUNATELY, GOES on. I attempted to put everything behind me and not focus on the second diagnosis that upended my life. I struggled to keep my mental health in check. I threw myself into social activities, masking the worry I felt inside. If they had missed the cancer once, who is to say it couldn't be missed again?

I spoke to Dr. Toussaint, who agreed with Dr. Gauthier: yet another "all clear" and no treatment on the horizon. Again, I was told to live my life and be happy. Easier said than done—and even harder to believe. I constantly worried that the cancer was deep inside of me, growing again. I met a breast cancer survivor, Sandra, who introduced me to her oncologist. I found myself across from yet another massive oak desk, pleading for assurance that I was actually okay this time. And again, I was told to live my life and be happy.

And so I tried. To the best of my ability.

My third and final (I hoped!) surgery was scheduled for January 2020. This would be the lipofilling surgery, the one that would make me happy with my breasts again. I pored over pictures online, excited about what the result could be. My mother booked her flight—she was a pro at solo international travel by now. She continued with her Duolingo in preparation for the trip. I had multiple presurgery appointments with Dr. Gauthier.

"I think you will have a very good result from the lipofilling," he said, as I stood topless in front of him with my hands on my hips, the breast cancer doctor's appointment stance. He took pictures and measured my breasts with his hands, jotting down notes. By this point, whipping off my top was a common occurrence for me.

"But what about the other breast? We can do a breast lift there and they'll both match better," he suggested.

I scrunched my face, not a fan of the idea. "I don't know. What would you do?" I asked.

"I would cut the areola and move the nipple up, and that would make the breast higher, have a higher effect." I looked down at my chest.

The truth was, I was really scarred from my many

surgeries. Every time a scalpel touched my body, it had resulted in ugly, raised keloids. I was happy with my other breast and I knew there was a strong possibility I could scar my beautiful, still-natural, all-American breast. I wasn't at all concerned about my breasts "not matching." The "not matching" and risk of secondary breast cancer concerns were something I had brought up when I requested a double mastectomy. For me, that ship sailed when I was rejected from having that surgery. But plastic surgeons are always concerned with perfection, even when it's unattainable.

"Well, I don't think I want that. I mean if you can do it *without* cutting me at all—some kind of way, then okay. But I do not want the other breast operated on," I said. Possibly a tall order, or even an impossible one, but I wanted to stick to my guns. My body was riddled with painful, itchy keloids, and the last thing I wanted was to add more for the sake of vanity.

"Okay, sure," he said. We settled up the paperwork, and I handed over a check for the surgery—one I pleaded with the receptionist not to cash until a couple months later. It was a trick I'd recently learned.

Weeks later, on January 14, 2020, I found myself again at the operating clinic—the one full of hot nurses and orderlies. I took three weeks off of work for this surgery, determined to recover better than I had in the past. In hindsight, I saw that my previous determination to go back to work as quickly as possible hadn't helped my recovery—

only my bosses. The same bosses who didn't seem to care one way or another that I was risking my health to appear like a model employee.

We went through the usual presurgery routine (this time I shaved myself beforehand), and I was wheeled away into the small operating theater for the third and final time. After this, life could truly begin.

I woke up in a small yellow room, across from a young Black man sitting at a computer. "*Hola,*" I said, the first word that came to mind, much to his confusion. What can I say, the anesthesia did a number on me. After much back-and-forth, I rolled down the hallway, back to my room, where my mother waited.

Dr. Gauthier sidled up to my bed in the doorway. "Hello—the surgery went well. They both look great," he said. My heart sank with the realization of his words. "They . . . both . . . ?" I asked incredulously. "Yep, they both look good," he responded. "I'll leave the paperwork with the nurses," he said and strolled off.

I looked down at my bandaged chest. I couldn't see or feel anything. My chest was bound so tightly that I couldn't tell what had been done. But I knew from his words that despite my asking him not to, he had operated on my other breast. Since my diagnosis, I had lost all agency over my body, but this was to a level I never expected. Not only were my wishes disregarded, but this was outright medical malpractice. They rolled me into the room where my mother was excited to see me. I immediately burst into tears.

I was just a passenger on this train. I wasn't making any of the decisions or even directing the conductor. And with this last surgery, my body autonomy was completely ruined. Not just my body autonomy, but my body as well.

Once I left the hospital and my bandages were removed, I saw what I already knew—I'd been operated on on both sides. And the pain I felt every day in one breast would now be in both.

9

Even the Most Beautiful City in the World Can Feel Like the Loneliest

I loved living in Paris, but I missed the feeling of community. In NYC, I had a big, wonderful, diverse community. I was active in my church in Harlem, my friends there gathering at each other's apartments for Bible study and meeting for picnics in the park. My work friends and I regularly met up at the Rink Bar at 30 Rock or a nearby Irish pub after particularly grueling days of breaking news. I had my core group of girlfriends who I saw nearly every weekend. When I was diagnosed with cancer, my friends Juli and Ola immediately bought plane tickets, coming to Paris that September to cheer me up and support me after my mastectomy. We took boat rides and made champagne toasts at the *Moulin Rouge*; they did everything they could to keep a smile on my face. My American community was legit—no other way to say it.

Moving to France meant finding a new community, almost starting from the ground up. My graduate program helped—I met and made many lifelong friends there. We enjoyed picnics on the *quai* of the Seine, lazy days drinking coffee and people-watching on café terraces, long walks crisscrossing the city, and even going to concerts like Cardi B at *Palais de Tokyo*.

But life in Paris is transient. Expats come and go often, leaving at the end of work contracts, leaving to help take care of family at home, or leaving because they couldn't find a job in the tight Paris job market. It was common to become good friends with someone and one or two years later they'd be gone, back to their home country. You'd have to find a new friend to fill the void. Even my school program had this problem. Out of my entire graduate cohort, fewer than ten people were able to stay in Paris long term. At one point, I went to going-away parties almost every week.

Even worse were the visiting Americans—you'd meet them at social events, where they explained that they "just moved to Paris" and needed friends. After enjoying their company and investing in the friendship, you'd find out they weren't actually living in Paris—they had moved for three months without a visa, just to say they'd lived abroad. They always reassured you that they'd come back with a visa, to build a new life in Paris—but that often never happened. They would be back in the US in just a few weeks, and you'd never see your newfound buddy ever again.

Americans have the stereotype of being extremely

friendly, and after moving to Paris, I see why. Penetrating the tight-knit French friendship circles felt impossible. French people are loyalists—it's not uncommon for them to be friends with the same people from childhood—and there's no space for anyone new unless you slide in as a romantic partner of one of them. The *crèche* (daycare) friends, as we like to call them, are harder to penetrate than Fort Knox. It also takes a lengthy amount of time to forge a friendship.

Whereas Americans will call you a friend after a few meetings, I remember going to numerous coffees and lunches with a French coworker and wondering, "Okay, when is this girl going to consider me a friend, because this is an intense vetting process?"

But once you're in, you're in. And you're a friend for life and lucky to have them.

I wasn't there yet.

More than just needing community, I needed support. After my diagnosis, I didn't know anyone my age with breast cancer—or cancer at all. I didn't know if the things I felt were normal or outrageous. I didn't know if I was doing enough or if I could have been doing more to get through the journey.

My attempts to find community online and in the US, at the bra shop, had all ended in a fail. Before my mastectomy, I had emailed a cancer support group based in France. They asked me to call them so we could speak—but in the flurry of preparations for the surgery, I never reached out. I received an email from them while still in my hospital bed after the mastectomy. "We haven't heard from you, so we assume you don't need our help anymore." Thanks for the "support," I guess. Disgusted, I promptly deleted the email.

Months later, I decided to try again: there must be some sort of help or support available. My late-night googling finally yielded results—there was a young adult cancer support group that met once a month over dinner.

◆ ◆ ◆

I LEFT WORK EARLY, SCURRYING out of the office shortly after five. I was determined to make it on time. Tonight, I'd go to the support group. I folded my hands over and over, eyes darting upward at the Métro map illuminating the stops, during the hour-long trek to the other side of the city.

I didn't spend much time in this part of the city—the 13th arrondissement of Paris. And when I did, it was mostly to eat at the abundance of delicious Chinese restaurants. My stomach was tied in knots, but I was ready to get some much-needed support and hopefully make new friends. My broken French aside, my mental health was in a precarious state. I was racked with anxiety most days and depression still lingered. I had started seeing a therapist after my diagnosis, but I knew I needed more. I had to at least try.

After getting off the train, I plodded down the poorly lit streets, the early November darkness having already descended upon Paris. I followed the Google Maps blue dot down residential streets until I approached a hospital complex, the app telling me I'd finally reached my destination.

The listed location of the support group was vague—all I had to go on was an address, no building or room number. Pushing through the gate, I roamed the hospital grounds, looking for this elusive room that held the support group.

I timidly walked the corridors of the hospital, too self-conscious about my broken French and too prideful to ask for help. Up one floor, down another, around one corner, and peeking into various rooms. After ten unfruitful minutes of searching, I paused at a nurse's station. I approached the man at the desk, at this point more than a little late for the group meeting.

"*Bonsoir, excusez-moi. Je cherche Madame Moreau?*" I asked, mentioning the leader of the support group. "*Comment?*" the man asked, frowning. I repeated my request, adding to please excuse my French and accent—hoping it would soften the man's response.

"I don't know what you're talking about," he barked in French, his voice booming throughout the packed waiting room. Bored patients in the waiting room turned their heads. In line behind me, people stretched their necks to see what the commotion was. Speaking louder when someone doesn't speak a language fluently is clearly an annoying worldwide response. As if I wasn't already self-conscious and nervous.

Thanking him, I ducked my head down and darted out of the hospital. I was over an hour away from my apartment and twenty minutes late for the meeting, and no one was around to help—or even wanted to.

I stood in the parking lot, considering my options, when

I remembered I had written down a phone number. Digging in my purse, I pulled out the number and placed the call as a last-ditch attempt. *"Bonjour ? Oui ?"* A woman's voice came alive on the line, deep and scratchy. I excitedly responded, but it became clear she couldn't understand my French and also didn't speak any English. Dejected, I crumpled to the curb and began to cry.

After dealing with cancer for almost a year, I realized the mental and emotional side effects of the disease had hit me—and hit me hard. I didn't take much time off work. I dealt with much of it by myself, while working a job that wasn't understanding—or even cognizant—of my situation. I always took so much pride in being strong, being the strong friend, the strong family member. The strong Black woman. I put it all on my shoulders as best as I could, so as to not bother or be a burden to anyone else. And in that moment, sitting on the curb in the dark hospital parking lot, I broke.

I broke because I'd gone through so much. I broke because I knew I was in a depression danger zone and I wanted help but, in this moment, it was impossible. I broke because all I wanted to do was express myself and be understood, and no one was willing to give that to me.

I didn't know what to do or where to go, so I called my friend Carmen. At this point, I was very late for the support group that I didn't even know would understand my story in my broken French.

Sobbing on the phone, tears and snot running down my face, I explained the situation to Carmen. She urged me to come to her place for dinner instead. Rising from the curb, ready to give up and go to her apartment in the 6th, I got a call on the other line. Madame Moreau called me back, and through slow and clear French in a raspy voice, she directed me back to the front door of a houselike building. As I approached the small building, Madame Moreau appeared like a vision, with a shock of red hair and large glasses, waving her arms at me to welcome me in.

It happened so quickly—from my parking-lot breakdown to finding Madame Moreau. Looking at her was like seeing an oasis in the desert. I felt seen by her. She didn't know me and went out in the street looking for me, to make sure I could join them. It was a foreign feeling for me in Paris. And when I followed her up the stairs where everyone else waited—looking around at the smiling and welcoming faces of strangers who all had one thing in common with me—I knew despite the language barrier and the troubles before, this was something I needed, more than I ever imagined.

The support group was young adult in name only: around the dinner table was a group of ten people of all ages and ethnicities. We were diverse in cancer too—there was ovarian, throat, stomach, and more. Madame Moreau laid out a spread—a healthy, home-cooked meal—with couscous, bread, dips, and salads, each loaded up with ingredients known for their cancer-fighting benefits. I dried my tears and listened to my new acquaintances recount their cancer journeys—and shed a few tears for them as well. Through their stories, I realized my feelings of solitude were not just because I was an expat dealing with cancer—these people were French, with families and long-standing communities, and they often felt alone on their journeys as well. They'd lost friends and jobs and their sense of self. Much like I had.

When it came time to recount my story, I did so in my elementary French, explaining my diagnosis and surgery. There was another American in the group, married to a Frenchwoman, so he piped up to help translate and smooth out my story. He helped me when I didn't understand some of the words in others' stories as well.

This support group was different from my foray into the online groups. It wasn't about getting all the information or the facts or even the science behind your diagnosis and treatment. It wasn't about placing blame on why you got this god-awful disease or scolding you for not praying enough. It was about giving voice to your story and knowing you're not the only one. I didn't feel overwhelmed or like I had to take up arms immediately against my cancer with alkaline water and essential oils—I felt understood.

At the end of the night, we wished each other well for upcoming treatments, surgeries, and scans. We *bised* goodbye, stomachs and hearts full. The support group wasn't what I'd expected, but it was exactly what I needed.

◆ ◆ ◆

IN ADDITION TO THE SUPPORT group, I got a cancer mentor. After selling my camera, the person I sold it to connected me with his business partner, a recent cancer survivor. He told me about an organization he worked with called Imerman Angels. "They match you with a cancer mentor, someone to help you on your journey," he said.

I'd had many mentors in my life—and had been one a time or two—but a cancer mentor? I reached out to the organization and was matched with Lauren. Based in New Jersey, she'd been through breast cancer just two years earlier. Although we were thousands of miles apart, she became my sounding board. I fired away my questions and concerns to her on WhatsApp, and she responded in long and thoughtful texts, calming my fears.

She understood—like me, she was young and single when diagnosed. She had the same fears and concerns that I did, but also the wisdom gained from being a few years removed from it. Lauren wasn't physically with me, but her presence was felt.

I was also growing my community in Paris, even with my lack of French friends. It surprised me how people you've only known for a year or two can step up when you're alone. After my last reconstructive surgery, my mother was surprised by all the friends who stopped by with gifts. They brought chocolate, flowers, guacamole—anything they could to lift my spirits.

Your friends easily become your family in expat communities. I couldn't remember the last time I'd visited a friend at home after surgery or in the hospital in the US—family, yes, but a friend? I'd be more likely to send flowers during a long day at the office, texting periodically to check in with them or giving them a call at the end of the day. My new friends even embraced my mother, adding her on WhatsApp, to keep her up to date once she flew home, and inviting her to dinners and picnics while she stayed in Paris.

My community in Paris looked wildly different from my community in NYC. It was less segregated and more diverse—a group of risk takers, people who left their home country for the unknown. People who speak more than one language, often more than two. I missed big American hugs, but my friends showed their love through baked goods, raucous dinner parties with home-cooked food, and *bises*.

So many of my graduate-school friends left Paris that I needed to continue growing my circle every chance I had. A happy hour invite? I was there. Dinner at a new restaurant? Count me in. I spent nearly every night a week at a social outing, which didn't account for all the coffees and lunches I had while at work.

I didn't realize then just how vital these growing friendships would be for what was up ahead.

10

This Is My Year

This is my year—at least that's what I thought. Both my breasts were in pain from the surgery, but it couldn't dim my hope. After two stressful years of dealing with breast cancer, physical and emotional pain, and tight finances, I was ready to start living my best life. My life had been on pause for the past two years—and my elevator had been going between the emergency stop button and the down button this entire time.

I watched as friends met their future husbands, got promotions and fancy new jobs, and started growing their families. None of that was happening for me—I was "just" fighting cancer. An achievement, yes, but not as sexy as the major moves everyone else made. But it was okay—as of January 2020, with my last surgery complete, the world would be my oyster.

I even had a new apartment—yes, apartment number five. I finally made it out of my fire/health/life-hazard apartment in the 16th and moved into a new place, a studio in the trendy Marais district. The owners, a set of siblings who inherited the apartment from their mother, told me they would be selling in 2022, so I could stay for three years. It seemed feasible to me. Hopefully, by 2022 I could buy a place of my own, something I had dreamed about for years.

No feeling like a second-rate citizen with a backdoor entrance. No spider-monkey crawling into bed. And most important, no cohabitating with multiple rodent roommates. It also had one of my new apartment requirements: a kitchen with a door. Easy to guess why that was added to my list.

The best part was the air conditioning. The apartment was fitted with a fancy heat-pump air conditioner. Every night I turned my place into an icebox and cozied under the blankets.

I made travel plans and plans to boost my professional network in Paris. I was going to hit the gym and slim down to my ideal weight. The year 2020 would be a big one for me: a new apartment, all done with surgeries, and now real life could truly commence. I wanted to make Paris my home—despite it all, I enjoyed the life I was building in the city. I would even start dating again in earnest. I could move forward with finding love.

◆ ◆ ◆

I HIGHLY IDENTIFIED WITH AUDRE Lorde when she wrote, "my primary concerns two days after mastectomy were hardly about what man I could capture in the future," but I still desired romantic love. Things with André hadn't worked out, but I felt I was ready now—ready to jump back in and find the man of my dreams. After the mastectomy and now the botched breast lift, however, I wasn't sure if love would be in the cards for me. Superficial standards exist in all cultures—do they weigh more heavily in France?

In France, the stigmas around being sexually active don't exist. Many a time, a Frenchman stared deeply into my eyes and told me, "It's just about a feeling." They could never explain what that meant, and it tended to be red flag number one. Often, sleeping together quickly was a required "chemistry test" to see if you were worth the time and effort.

For me, dating in France seemed arguably more physically focused than in America, which is a horrifying realization when you've gone through breast cancer. Not to say I would be sleeping with any of the men—I wouldn't—but if the physical is such a crucial aspect of the initial dating process, then why would anyone stick around after finding out I'm lacking a big portion of what attracts many of them in the first place? In a world where people strive to look "Instagram perfect"—from using filters to knowing your angles—with my set of botched boobs, I now felt like damaged goods.

After my almost year-long sabbatical from dating after breaking it off with André, I redownloaded my old frenemies—the dating apps. Tinder, Hinge, Bumble, the works. I hated the gamification of dating, but there appeared to be no other option to meet your soulmate in France. I uploaded new pics of myself, trying to boost my confidence—after all, confidence is sexy, right? I paid special attention to make sure my chest appeared symmetrical in my outfits and my scars were hidden. But no matter what, I only attracted men who were not ready, were playing games, or in general were not a good option.

After my third and final reconstructive surgery, in January 2020, I swiped on Daniel. Daniel was a full-lipped, gorgeous Martiniquais, with a charm I fell for immediately. He was a talented musician, photographer, and faithful meditator who made me laugh. His English was lilted with a slight Caribbean accent. We would spend all day and night texting each other, going from deep conversations to movie discussions and cracking jokes. He was smart, charming, and didn't take himself too seriously—something I didn't find often in the French dating scene.

"Robin—he's a whole snack! I didn't think he would be that cute," said my best friend after looking at the pictures I forwarded. "He's way better-looking than most of the guys you've dated, by far," she proclaimed. Only a best friend (and your mom) can pump you up and shade you at the same time. Either way, it made me more excited for the date and to see how he measured up in person.

I met him in a café in République for our first date—a tiny, crowded restaurant where we perched on barstools. I showed up in a leather miniskirt, with an oversized sweater big enough to hide the medical corset I was wearing while recovering from the lipofilling surgery just a week earlier. Despite it all, I felt it was important to get out there. If there's one thing that a single woman in her thirties constantly hears in the twenty-first century, it's to "Get out there!" I was just doing my duty, making an effort.

When I laid eyes on Daniel, he was even more attractive in person. This would definitely be a good date, I thought. Throughout the evening, we talked about everything from our travels to our family to our dating history. We were vibing. The noise of the café fell away, and all we could see was each other. Inevitably, the convo turned to differences between France and the US, namely healthcare.

"So, what do you think about healthcare here? Americans always like the healthcare," he prompted with a smirk, sipping his beer. "I like the healthcare here—it's different from the US, but the level of care is high, in my opinion. I spent five days in the hospital and it didn't break the bank," I responded. "You were in the hospital for several days? What, did you get a boob job?" he cracked.

I immediately went cold. Up to this point, the date had been going well. We'd ordered another round, his body leaned in close toward me, and my legs crossed, brushing his knee. It's official—we're into each other. But this was a fork in the road. I didn't know if I should take the chance and mention my medical history—it did come up organically— or do I deflect deflect deflect and possibly scare him off?

I twirled my straw and laughed nervously, trying to decide which path to take. "Well, actually, yeah. I did get a boob job. I had breast cancer and had a mastectomy," I replied, trying to keep as much lightness in my voice as possible, despite my heart beating out of my chest.

"Are you okay now? How is your health?" Daniel responded, leaning in, his brow furrowed in concern. Okay, great, I thought, he's not appalled or shirking away in horror. "Well, I just had surgery last week, so I'm still recovering a bit—which is why my mom was in town." I explained to him everything I had been through, and he listened attentively. Maybe this would work out after all.

Our first date ended with him walking me home—a long, romantic walk through the city past midnight. I was over the moon. After such a harrowing two years, maybe I was finally turning a corner to get my happy ending. Premature much? Definitely. The cart was way ahead of the horse and around the corner. By the time he planned dinner and a movie for our third date, it seemed like we were well on our way to being exclusive. Before you say I was jumping the gun, though, hear me out.

Dating in France is different from dating in NYC. In NYC, you can date a guy for eight months and he'll say, "We're just 'talking.'"

In France, by the first kiss or third date, you're considered exclusive. Too many times I explained to men, "Yes, I understand that's the French way, but I'm American. I'd prefer to get to know you a bit more before we commit."

Our third date was planned and I looked forward to it—but it seemed like I was the only one. I noticed a shift in his energy—his texts became infrequent and cold. The long, engaging text threads that originally hooked me became few and far between. So much so, I asked him several times if he wanted to reschedule or cancel. "I'm fine, I'm fine, let's go," he assured me.

When he arrived at the movie theater for the Star Wars showing, my intuition was right. But maybe it had nothing to do with me at all. Daniel was glum, low energy, and disinterested. I wasn't feeling well—my chest still hurt from my most recent surgery—but I put on a big smile and hoped the date could be salvaged.

Over dinner, it was obvious I'd been right all along. "Okay, what's really going on here? What's the deal?" I asked as he pushed his food around on his plate. He sat up and pushed his plate back. "You're not seducing me at all. There's no seduction coming from you," he explained.

I tilted my head and crossed my arms over my chest. Sharp nerve pain pricked my reconstructed breasts and dull aches cramped in my stomach, back, and chest. I was buttoned up in the world's tightest medical corset from the surgery two weeks prior (which he knew about) and dolled up in heels (on cobblestones), while sitting across from a man who told me his issue with me is that I'm not seducing him.

I wish I could say I grabbed my purse and walked out without saying a word. But I didn't. What I didn't do was try to change his mind. I looked him up and down and crossed my legs. I glanced to the left and right in the now emptying café before leaning back in my chair.

"So you mean to tell me, first and foremost, you believe it's my role to seduce you and that I'm not doing such, when you know I am actively recovering from surgery?"

He doubled down, nodding in agreement with everything I said. It was incredible how quickly things turned. You have to give it to him—he decided to lean all the way into being a jerk.

"So are you saying you just want to be friends?" I asked, trying to lead him to the path of redemption. I gave him his out, but slouched at the table, he only responded with a one-shoulder shrug. I gathered my things, paid my portion of the bill, and walked out.

I marched the five blocks home, occasionally wobbling on the cobblestones in my four-inch heels. We'd only been on three dates, but I was devastated. I had put too much weight on our brief courtship—and he was not the person I thought he was. I gave him more grace than he extended me.

I felt like I would never find a man who would understand my journey, my ordeal. I was scared that maybe I had just walked out on my last shot. I went back to my studio apartment and cried myself to sleep. I was so tired. Tired of having to try so hard. I just needed things to go my way for once. I needed a moment of calm.

◆ ◆ ◆

LIFE POSTSURGERY AND POST-DANIEL WASN'T as calm as I'd hoped. From my studio in the Marais, I began reading a headline here and there about a virus in China. My interest in international news is what brought me to Paris, and that interest didn't wane once I moved. Perusing the news, I saw the reports start as a small mention, then the virus appeared more frequently—and with more details and an increasing number of sick patients. In my area, a section of the Marais with a large Asian population, I noticed my neighbors buying and wearing surgical masks. Grocery stores were full of shoppers, stocking up on essentials, a few of them wearing masks.

I'm not a doomsday prepper—honestly, how can you be in a tiny Parisian apartment anyway?—but I am observant. As the number of masked neighbors picked up, I set out to find my own protection, without any luck. Pharmacies were sold out, as they said on signs on the door written in Mandarin and Cantonese.

Outside of my neighborhood, life in Paris seemed to be completely normal. Most of Paris—most of the world—seemed to not take notice of what was occurring in China. Under strict orders to not carry anything heavy after my surgery, I took several trips a week to the grocery store to buy as many canned goods and toilet paper rolls as I could carry.

As a recent breast cancer survivor, the thought of getting ill again kept me up at night. The health anxiety I hoped would vanish returned but with a different villain. Riding the Métro, I would hear a cacophony of coughs and sneezes. No one covered their mouths, and during rush hour I was mere inches away from their faces. I curbed my outings, staying home more often than not. The thought of riding the Métro could make my stomach churn. My anxiety was at an all-time high. In the years past, getting sick meant possibly delaying my surgeries or causing complications. Now, contracting the virus meant I could die.

Dealing with cancer gave me post-traumatic stress disorder—and not just me: studies show about eighty percent of breast cancer survivors suffer from PTSD post-diagnosis. The sleepless nights were back, but this time I was worrying that the cancer could return. Or I tossed and turned, remembering the days before cancer, wondering if I somehow could have caught it earlier, would I still have my breasts? The fear and anxiety were debilitating. I feared death, knowing it could have easily come for me, whereas I never did before. And this novel, spreading virus triggered many of these feelings tenfold.

In late February, I contacted my human resources manager and asked if I could work from home. "I just don't feel comfortable going into the office, because something is going around and I just had surgery. I know myself, my body—I'm not at one hundred percent to fight any type of illness," I said. They agreed, but I could tell they felt it was a bit dramatic.

Things began to shut down—slowly at first, and then quickly like a hammer. While sipping coffee in a café with a colleague, we heard screams erupting outside in the bustling *Les Halles* shopping center. "University is closed!" teenagers shouted, running to spread the news. The next day, the news was not as joyous, as bars, nightclubs, and movie theaters—and, worst of all, restaurants—closed.

Everything took a sharp dive on March 16, when President Emmanuel Macron announced we would be going into a two-week lockdown—unable to leave our homes for work, social outings, or anything at all really. He said we were in "a war" with coronavirus. We could go outside only to get groceries or walk our dogs.

Many Parisians fled to the countryside, preferring to ride out the lockdown in a more comfortable fashion. Friends flew back to the US, booking flights as quickly as they could to go back to the comfort of home—where there wasn't yet a lockdown and they could live life as normal. With the fear of the unknown, it was easier to be with your family.

As the number of cases and deaths rose in France, I didn't even consider flying back to the US. Through the ups and downs, Paris was still my home and—most important—my doctors were here. Plus, it was too risky to fly back and possibly pick up the virus en route and bring it to my parents. I still worried about not being there for my family—or them contracting the virus elsewhere and never being able to see them again.

But as much as I love and worry for my family, repatriating for an undetermined amount of time while still paying rent on my apartment and possibly losing my job wasn't an option. I could get stuck in the US and my residency card could expire—making it harder to come back. My work contract was up for renewal, and I needed to see things through. Plus, I trusted the French healthcare system—for better or for worse, it was the system that had saved my life not so long ago.

Two weeks of lockdown turned into three weeks. Then four weeks. Then five weeks. I planted myself in front of the TV for each presidential address. *"Chers compatriotes,"* Macron always began. In WhatsApp groups, friends would send alerts about upcoming press conferences or addresses, speculating on what the message would be.

I watched Olivier Véran and Edouard Philippe, the health minister and prime minister, at daily press conferences, hoping for an announcement of the end of lockdown. Instead, we learned how many people were dying. Trains—mostly out of use due to our inability to travel—were converted into traveling hospitals, transporting the ill. We learned when France would receive more masks—there was a nationwide shortage. There was a shortage of antibacterial gel as well. I learned to make my own via YouTube, while the winemakers and luxury companies such as LVMH stepped up to try to fill the gap.

I refreshed my Chrome tab on the Johns Hopkins Covid-19 map several times a day, seeing where France fell in the ranking of illnesses and deaths. France, a country the size of Texas with a population of only sixty-six million, seemed to be losing the war against Covid.

As the numbers increased not only in France but in Europe too, my anxiety turned to fear—a controllable fear. If I stayed in my four-hundred-square-foot studio, about the size of a two-car garage (they're getting bigger each time!), I would be safe. With the lockdown, I was allowed to go grocery shopping but decided against it. I ordered my groceries online, dutifully wearing gloves and wiping them down with bleach wipes after each delivery.

I didn't see anyone. I buzzed in the delivery men and

instructed them to set the groceries outside my door. I only opened my door once I heard the elevator door close and saw the hallway was empty. One day while I was disinfecting my groceries in the hallway, a neighbor stepped out with her baby—I'm not sure who was happier to see a different face, me or the baby.

Thanks to Covid-19, the Marais studio wore many hats. It was my home, my office, my happy-hour spot, my restaurant, and my gym. The eighth-floor studio had a tiny balcony for outdoor space, but it was completely unusable due to aggressive pigeons who decided it was their home (what was with me and animals taking over my apartment?).

Gazing out my eighth-floor window was the only way I could lay eyes on another person. I watched my neighbor—a man across the street—having his daily coffee on his balcony and tending to his rosebushes. Being on a high floor with an unusable balcony meant I couldn't see anything but him and the sky. Not the street, not the sidewalk, nothing at all.

The silence was deafening. There were no cars zooming down the normally busy *Rue Beaubourg*, no chatter from groups of friends walking down the street. No planes leaving their chemtrails overhead in the sky. Sometimes the silence was broken by rhythmic clops of horses marching down my street. I couldn't see them—of course, I couldn't see *anything*—but I wondered just what *was* happening out there in the new normal. It was eerie.

As vigilant as I was, many people cut corners as much as they could, so they could have some semblance of a regular life. A lockdown in Parisian apartments was far different from the ones my friends in the US would experience a few weeks later. Most people resided in minuscule apartments without any outdoor space. People gathered in their apartment courtyards to socialize with neighbors without the watchful eye of the police, who would hand out fines to rule-breakers.

If you had a pet, you had some relief. You were allowed to go out to walk your pet, but only within a certain kilometer distance. Some dogs had never been walked so much in their lives. Singles coordinated "first dates" in grocery stores—chatting on Tinder and arranging to meet in an aisle at their local Carrefour, within the approved radius.

I even booted up my Tinder again, hoping to find someone to chat with while sitting in my apartment for days on end.

I started talking to Nicolas, a burly Italian man with the smoothest radio voice. Think Barry White, but Italian. We spent hours exchanging voice messages—him from his apartment in the 9th and me from my apartment in the 3rd. We were less than a kilometer away but unable to meet due to the strict regulations of our lockdown.

We made plans to meet once the lockdown was lifted—although I wasn't physically attracted to him, personality and kindness ranked high on my list, now more than ever. But during a deep conversation, I opened up about my battle with breast cancer. He pondered what I said, carefully choosing his next words. He said his mother battled breast cancer—and died from it. I felt my heart opening up, feeling that maybe it wasn't too soon to tell someone and that he would be someone who understood.

Then I never heard from him again. At least we never met—an upside to the lockdown, I suppose.

But Tindering wasn't all I did during the lockdown. I tried to remain fit, running up and down the stairs in my apartment building to stay active. I took zinc and vitamin C pills—the rumor mill said they helped—and did breathing exercises to increase my lung capacity. Every night at 7 p.m., I went to my kitchen window to clap for the first responders.

I baked, an activity I had loved in the US but hadn't tackled in France. I made cheesecake brownies and a delicious lemon loaf—until my scratchy throat alerted me to a citrus intolerance. I downloaded an app to learn how to do a split, stretching in the only free space I had, next to the bed.

Friends and family pushed me to go outside to take in some fresh air and walk around the block. I didn't think it was worth it. I had just come out of a life-threatening illness with the best possible outcome, so why tempt fate?

Being far from my family during this scary period was difficult, but FaceTime and Zoom eased the loneliness. We video-chatted as much as we could and started a Sunday evening FaceTime get-together, laughing and playing Heads Up until 1 a.m. Paris time. During the week, I toasted with friends on virtual happy hours (I always included wine in my grocery delivery—it's France!).

My fear of falling ill was one I'd had since my 2018 diagnosis—but now the rest of the world felt it as well. As terrible as this sounds, it made me feel less alone. It wasn't just me who worried about my health at all times, and it wasn't just me who couldn't go out and live life in the sun. It was comforting to have everyone in the same mental and emotional space I'd felt for so long—everyone was experiencing a "pause" at the same time. No one was missing out on anything—we were all in it together.

In April, a few days before my thirty-sixth birthday, President Macron addressed the nation again. I hoped he would lift the lockdown so I could celebrate my birthday. Instead, he encouraged everyone to not cancel their doctor's appointments during the lockdown. Life was still happening, so people were continuing to fall ill in other ways—and skipping their medical appointments didn't help. Just a month earlier, I had emailed my oncologist to postpone a checkup—walking into a hospital during the height of the Covid-19 pandemic was not appealing to me. We would reschedule when the lockdown lifted, which, as just announced, would be in May.

◆ ◆ ◆

EIGHT WEEKS. EIGHT WEEKS OF solitude were finally over.

On May 11, I stepped outside my apartment building, something I hadn't done in eight weeks. The air smelled clean from the reduction of car and cigarette pollution. The sunshine grazed my face like a warm kiss. I would never take this for granted again. Exiting the building, both my shelter and prison, I felt like a butterfly emerging from a cocoon. Okay, less beautiful than that, more like a moth. There, that's more like it.

After eight intense weeks of lockdown, I truly believed—hoped, even—the pandemic was on its way behind us. The number of cases was going down. I called an Uber, mask pulled tightly across my face, and rode to my friend Isabelle's apartment for my first human contact in over two months. It was obvious life wouldn't be the same again for a long time—maybe even forever—but to finally be out in the sun and in my friend's warm embrace was needed. Hopefully, I could reunite with my family—either in August for summer vacation or in December for Christmas. We had all made it thus far without getting sick, and I was ready to get my life back on track.

During the lockdown, my job had offered me a new contract, one with more stability. My visa was set to expire in October, but thanks to the new contract, I would have a renewal on the way. To process the new contract, I had to complete a medical exam—an update of the one I did when I originally joined the company. A few days after the end of the lockdown, I headed to Dr. Burton, my generalist, for a physical.

Dr. Burton was one of my favorite doctors. A stylish British woman with an impeccably cut blonde bob. With her looks, she could have easily been an actress. She was always chicly dressed in a uniform of a crisp button-down with a silk scarf. I felt underdressed for our appointments. But above all, she was attentive and thorough with a great sense of humor and spunk. When I once told her about a comment a coworker made about an upcoming reconstructive surgery, she responded, "Oh, I bet if it was about his *balls* he'd suddenly find more empathy." I knew I could run to her with any issue and she'd do her best to find a solution for me—even holistic ones. She had my back, no matter the problem.

It was bizarre going to the doctor postlockdown. I walked sixty minutes to her *Parc Monceau* office, masking up quickly when I came in close contact with others. I was avoiding the Métro, but I was sweating like a pig in the heat.

I sat on the exam table, mask on, facing Dr. Burton. She did a thorough physical, working her way through the checklist my job required. The idea of doing a physical before starting a new position always gave me the jitters—why was my health monitored for me to make a living? If something was found, did that mean I would lose my job?

Dr. Burton finished up the physical by checking my vitals and conducting a breast exam. "Everything looks good," she said, jotting down notes. "Oh, wait—I checked your right breast, but I forgot to check the other one. I mean, you had a mastectomy; I'm sure it's fine."

She began the pitter-patter movements with her fingers, around the top and sides of my breasts, then my armpit. "Hmm," she murmured, massaging my armpit. "What is it?" I asked. "I feel a lump here—have you felt this before?" I pressed my fingers into my left armpit, slightly above a long, ridged scar from my previous surgeries. "No, I haven't," I said, which was true. In my previous surgery, so many lymph nodes were taken out that I never really touched my armpit. Not to mention, I still had no feeling there, so I tended to avoid it—barely shaving it—to make sure I wouldn't accidentally injure myself.

"Well, I'm sure it's fine, but let's just get another look at that, okay? I'll write you up something for a sonogram," she said. I took the prescription and left her office. I'd started so many new routines during the lockdown: exercise programs, armpit exfoliations, whatever I could do to stave off boredom. For once, I wasn't worried or anxious. I was certain the lump was just a result of a new routine—and the tests would confirm my hunch.

11

The Carousel of Cancer

The movie *Groundhog Day* was a blockbuster when it came out in 1993, and the cultural reference has lasted for decades. For those who don't know, in the movie, Bill Murray's life is stuck in a loop—every single day the same, with the same things happening over and over and over again. It's a trope that's since been used in plenty of TV shows and movies, Netflix's *Russian Doll* being one of them.

My life was now Groundhog Day.

Once again, just like two years earlier in 2018, June and July were filled with endless testing. The week after my appointment with Dr. Burton, I found myself topless with my arms raised in a sonogram room.

The doctor handed me a paper towel to wipe my armpit free from the sticky sonogram lubricant. *"Je ne sais pas ce que c'est, mais—" "S'il vous plaît, en anglais,"* I interrupted. My French had improved due to my daily lockdown French classes, but for something so important, I needed to be able to understand completely. "I can't tell what the lump is," he said, continuing in English. "The sonogram isn't clear. You'll have to talk to your doctor about it." I took my scans and moved on to the next set of tests.

My doctors ran two blood tests—not an easy feat for someone like me, with hidden veins. The bloodwork seemed fine. My CA 125 and CA 15.3 numbers—the cancer antigen markers that doctors monitor if they suspect cancer—were completely normal. But the lump stayed there—not getting smaller, but also not getting bigger.

Just like in 2018, my fingers would find their way to the lump, this time in my armpit, and begin pressing and massaging. Wondering. I was beginning to wonder if it was all just an allergic reaction to detoxing my armpits, or some other terrible thing I had done out of boredom during the lockdown. Dr. Toussaint, my oncology surgeon, prescribed a biopsy of the lump—which we now assumed was a swollen lymph node—to make sure we weren't missing anything.

I breathed a sigh of relief when he emailed my results: the biopsy showed no sign of cancer cells.

Throughout the weeks of testing, the lump remained. I pressed on it with my fingers during my showers, hoping pressure could flatten it. Meanwhile, life in Paris was starting to feel normal again: restaurants were open, and we could do more socializing than just meeting in parks.

I went to a friend's place for a Bastille Day gathering, watching the fireworks from her balcony with an Eiffel Tower view. "I'm beginning to be afraid everything is going to blow up again," I said, gazing at fireworks illuminating the sky and cradling my champagne flute. "Don't worry about it—I'm sure it's just swollen from an infection, or maybe the chemicals you used during exfoliation—I'm sure you'll be fine," she insisted. I hoped she was right. I didn't want to survive a pandemic just to be taken out by cancer. I held on to her words tightly. Going through another cancer battle was unimaginable. I had already been through so much.

The biopsy results didn't satisfy Dr. Toussaint. He prescribed a PET scan, a highly complex (and expensive) scan that shows "metabolic" areas in your body. Shaped like a donut, it's used to diagnose cancer and to find cancer cells anywhere in the body. For example, if someone's existing cancer had spread or if their chemo treatment wasn't working, the metabolic areas would show in bright colors on the scan. There were various noncancerous reasons an area could light up as well—inflammation and fibroids, to name a couple. I'd never had one done before. If the lymph node was cancerous, then the PET scan would definitely show it, and I'd light up like a Christmas tree.

The lymph node lit up, but the PET scan results were inconclusive.

After all the testing, there was still no definitive answer. I appreciated my doctors were being thorough, but if so many tests couldn't conclusively show I had cancer, surely it must be a good thing. I was still stuck in the cycle of testing—my personal Groundhog Day—but if it meant I would have peace of mind, that my doctors would have peace of mind, it would be worth it in the end.

Dr. Toussaint emailed me after the PET scan.

"The lymph node is still hypermetabolic, and we think it should be removed, to be certain it is benign," he said. I was surprised that after a sonogram, biopsy, blood tests, and PET scan, my doctors wanted to go one step further.

It seemed excessive, but I didn't have complaints. I trusted my doctors while noting the huge difference between my care in France and how I would be handled in the US. In the US, where health insurance companies are king, there's no way my insurance would have allowed me to go through so many tests. Not out of concern for my health—out of concern for their pockets. After a negative biopsy, my insurance in the US would likely refuse to pay for additional testing. The PET scan alone costs an average of seven thousand dollars nationwide. US health insurance likes to keep you on a budget—paying thousands to check and double-check seemed out of the budget.

Thankfully, my out-of-pocket costs and reimbursements weren't an issue this time around either. Due to the lockdown, I didn't spend much money and was able to pay upfront costs fairly easily. My finances had finally balanced out. My job had also changed my insurance with my new contract—my new insurance plan was completely private, and I no longer had to wait six weeks or more for meager reimbursements. Now the reimbursements were fast and close to one hundred percent of the cost.

Just like in 2018, I was glad I didn't have to jump through hoops, delaying testing, to gain insurance approval. I was able to get my tests done fairly quickly even during a full-fledged pandemic. Part of that was due to using a private hospital like the American Hospital—although the hospital took on their fair share of Covid cases, the public hospitals took the bulk of them—but also insurance worked differently in France. And for that, I was glad. Answers were coming, sooner rather than later.

I scheduled the surgery for the earliest date, just three weeks later. I was scared. Covid numbers were still in the thousands, and people were dying every day. Going to the hospital for my tests made me anxious—having surgery during Covid flat-out made me afraid.

◆ ◆ ◆

DEALING WITH MEDICAL TESTS WASN'T the only problem in the summer of 2020. In May 2020, the world watched as George Floyd Jr. was murdered by police officers in Minneapolis, Minnesota. Four thousand miles away, in my apartment in Paris, I sat on my bed and cried.

In the midst of a global pandemic, in which thousands of people are dying each day, racism takes no days off. They still find ways to kill us.

It was devastating to witness, especially with everything else happening in the world. I began watching CNN day and night, following the protests springing up in America, and then worldwide. Even in France. Paris had a reputation in America as being a haven for African Americans over the years, from James Baldwin to Josephine Baker. But France has its own fraught history with racism and police brutality—and the African American experience is not the end all be all.

Adama Traoré, a twenty-four-year-old Black Frenchman, died in police custody in July 2016, just outside of Paris. Traoré was pinned to the ground during his arrest, much like George Floyd, and went into physical distress immediately after. He was declared dead one hour after his arrest.

His sister, Assa Traoré, immediately leaped into action, fighting for justice for her brother. She started the Committee for Justice and Truth for Adama, organizing protests around Paris and using the rallying cry *"Justice pour Adama."* The surge in coverage of Black Lives Matter in America helped shine a light on her cause and to get the police officers involved arrested for her brother's death.

French people of all races and ages took to the streets in protest, chanting *"Justice pour Adama"* and "Black Lives Matter" alternately. American expats joined in, feeling helpless about the situation back home but glad to promote the cause in their adopted home of France.

I didn't feel comfortable going to the protests during a Covid wave—masks were still in short supply. French protests often ended in tear gas, once those without pure intentions showed up. I watched the protests on social media, shared links to show support, and found ways to help on my own. But there was a sense of unity among the Black people in France that I hadn't felt before. It wasn't about where you grew up, what language you spoke, or your background.

The history of race relations in France is complicated and didn't start with 2020. In 1998, when France won the

World Cup, the team was nicknamed *"Black Blanc Beur"* (Black, White, Arab) in celebration of the team's diversity. The celebration seemed short lived when just four years later, National Front, the far-right political party, advanced to the second round of presidential elections.

The 2020 protests weren't the first racial reckoning in France. In October 2005, the police-involved deaths of two Muslim teenagers, Zyed Benna and Bouna Traoré, sparked three weeks of unrest, first in their suburb of Clichy-sous-Bois and then across France. Nearly ten years later, the police officers in question were acquitted of failure to assist a person in danger.

I didn't move to France because I thought it was a magical place without racism, where I would be free to thrive in my Black Girl Magic. That never crossed my mind when choosing France. Living in France, I'd had my fair share of "Was this person racist to me or just rude?"—even more than I did in the US.

Incidents ranged from being ignored and dismissed to being refused tables at cafés to more blatant actions: a stranger insulting me at work, intimating that I'm uneducated, and multiple coworkers grabbing my braids like I'm a zoo animal. I guess Solange's "Don't Touch My Hair" wasn't a hit over here.

I even walked into a dinner party where someone proclaimed, "There's the chocolate lady." The minute I sat down, she asked to touch my hair. And no, they were not talking about eating chocolate prior to me walking in. Believe me, I asked.

The microaggressions are in abundance here, even though many non-POC French people would scoff and tell you, "France is not like America—don't bring that 'wokeism' over here." Some even touted the "benefits" of colonization. France has a race problem, whether they choose to acknowledge it or not. The history may not be the same as the US, but the difference in the root of the problem doesn't mean there *is* no problem.

And it was easy for some not to acknowledge it. France is one of the most diverse countries in Europe, but there's no data to bolster the claim. It's illegal in France to collect data based on race and ethnicity—a policy that was put in place after the horrors of World War II. There's no record of how many people of color live in France, which means there's no way to measure equality and equity in terms of housing, healthcare, education, or anything at all.

Through *Justice pour Adama* and the international Black Lives Matter movement, I hoped people were starting to see that France wasn't the racial utopia many Americans made it out to be.

The charged climate in France with Covid and BLM/police brutality protests made me feel selfish to have to focus on myself. But hopefully, once the surgery was done, I wouldn't need to.

◆ ◆ ◆

AND EVEN WITH EVERYTHING ELSE going on—it always came back to apartment musical chairs. In April 2020, during the lockdown, my landlords informed me they would be selling the apartment at the end of the year and that I needed to leave. Remember "we'll sell in 2022, so you can stay here for three years"? Well, I remembered it, but apparently they didn't. Buyers began visiting the apartment while I stood in the corner in my mask, like a fly on the wall. One potential buyer asked me to be honest about any problems in the apartment. My honesty led to him sneering in disgust at the owners and walking out on the sale.

Big surprise: the owners decided to offer me two months rent-free if I left as soon as possible. That wasn't my goal, but it was a good side effect.

We were still at the height of the pandemic, and the borders were closed. It ended up working in my favor: thousands of tourist rental apartments were sitting empty with no end in sight. Through a chance encounter at a Zoom birthday party, I met a woman who led me to my next place: apartment number six, a spacious one-bedroom in the 9th arrondissement, near the *Moulin Rouge*. I was making my way throughout the city.

I had always wanted to live in the 9th—it was on the list of qualities I coveted in a dream apartment. In fact, everything about the apartment was on that list. After so much apartment drama, I had manifested the perfect place. It had high ceilings with ornate crown molding, light crossing through the apartment with windows on all sides—even one in the bathroom. This apartment was much bigger than my former digs had been as well. No more apartments the size of a parking space—this was the size of a three-car garage. I was moving on up! It was owned and renovated by an Irish couple who'd lived in the US, so they had included all kinds of American-style touches like a washer and dryer. Having a dryer in France was like winning the lottery.

Like my previous place, the owners said they planned to take back the apartment in 2023, once they retired. But I would be all good until then. Maybe my luck was turning around—maybe the tests would come back clear, and I'd have a beautiful apartment to live my best life in.

I moved into the apartment two weeks before my scheduled surgery. I hoped it was a good omen.

◆ ◆ ◆

BACK AT THE AMERICAN HOSPITAL for another surgery—and my Covid anxiety was at an all-time high. Being in a hospital during a pandemic seemed counteractive to all my precautions to stay Covid-free. It wasn't my idea of a good time, not in the slightest.

Going to the hospital for my surgery this time was so different from the first. There were still a few similarities. It was a hot July day, much like the day of my mastectomy, almost the exact same day two years earlier. But there were no friendly faces to calm my nerves this time—the smiles were hidden behind masks.

But the biggest difference was that I was alone. Covid had closed the borders, and my family was unable to be by my side for this surgery. With only three weeks' notice, there was no way for them to get through the administrative drama required to attempt to come. I would have to go under the knife without them.

Without my family around, my friends stepped up. Lyneka had moved back to the US a year earlier, so she wasn't able to offer her support and fantastic note-taking skills this time around. But Carmen offered to come with me to the hospital—saying even if I didn't need anything physically, she'd be there for emotional support, which I appreciated. The surgery triggered feelings in me—feelings I thought were deeply buried. My mastectomy wasn't that long ago—so much had changed since then, but it was a mere two years ago. This lymph node surgery was already my second surgery of 2020—six months after my "final" surgery in January.

Carmen quickly became one of my closest friends in Paris, after meeting at a party in a coworker's apartment. While everyone stood around drinking wine and talking, we were the only ones tearing up the makeshift dance floor to the hip-hop/Latin mix. We danced breathlessly to everything from Daddy Yankee to Jay-Z, stopping only to say, "This is my song," before dancing even harder. During a dance break, she mentioned she brought (and had made) the popular guacamole at the party, and I was sold.

From there, our friendship grew with workplace coffees, long walks home, and Mexican-Chinese fusion dinners at her apartment with her Asian American husband. We weren't friends during my first battle with cancer, but she was there for me once we became friends—even taking my hysterical phone call from the hospital parking lot a year earlier. If I couldn't have my family with me for the surgery, she was the next best thing.

It was an outpatient surgery this time, no five-day stay in the Four Seasons–like hospital. I would be back in my apartment by evening, and Carmen promised me we would go out and celebrate the good news after. Restaurants had reopened in Paris one month earlier, and we could take advantage of the plentiful outdoor tables.

Walking into the American Hospital, I expected it to look like a war zone—a medic tent in the middle of a crisis. Doctors yelling "stat!" and gurneys barreling down the hallway. People coughing and spewing germs like the infamous Ebola virus movie theater scene in *Outbreak*, and oxygen tanks being rushed to hospital rooms. Families wailing and tossing themselves on the bodies of their loved ones. Maybe I watched too many movies, but it was my first pandemic—and hopefully my only. I had no idea what I was walking into. But it wasn't like that at all.

There were masks and hand gel everywhere, but I saw many noses hanging over masks—surprising, considering the location. It was eerily quiet—quieter than normal. It seemed true that people weren't going to the hospital for other medical issues anymore. Everyone stayed away out of fear, a luxury I didn't have. I rubbed my hands over and over in the hospital bed, waiting to be taken away. My face was sweating beneath my mask but I didn't want to risk taking it off. Carmen tried to distract me as I waited for an hour, then two, to be whisked away to the operating room.

After my two-hour wait, I was retrieved by a handsome

blond orderly (confirming again my theory on good-looking French healthcare workers). How did I know he was handsome? He was unmasked. I sped down the hallways in a wheelchair, pushed by the young, unmasked orderly. My friend had a theory that the more attractive you are, the less likely you are to wear your mask, so maybe he was right. Why cover a masterpiece?

One more time, for what I hoped was one last time, I cleared my mind and focused on pleasant thoughts of my family vacations in Delaware. And then I counted backward from ten as they injected the anesthesia.

◆ ◆ ◆

STILL DROWSY FROM THE ANESTHESIA, I was rolled down the hallway in a wheelchair, this time, unfortunately, not by the hot unmasked orderly. Maybe he was getting disciplined for his Covid hygiene, but more likely, he was just busy elsewhere in the hospital. After settling back into my room, they told me Dr. Toussaint would be stopping by to speak with me and give me the biopsy results of the lymph nodes. Carmen worked on her laptop in the corner, and I dozed off some of the anesthesia in my system to the soft clicking of her typing.

Dr. Toussaint strode into the room, pinching his mask firmly on his nose. We exchanged pleasantries and I introduced him to Carmen. "We took out two lymph nodes and they both tested positive for cancer. You have to do chemotherapy and then radiation. We can make an appointment with Dr. Reneau, the oncologist," he said.

"Wait—wait," I said, my eyes filling rapidly with tears. "What?" I screeched. "Can you slow down; this is a lot." Everything seemed to move too quickly, like fast-forward on a TV remote. Nothing made sense.

He inhaled slowly and began again. "The two lymph nodes we took out are cancerous, so we'll have to do further treatment. Most likely chemotherapy and radiation," he repeated. I looked down at my hands. I looked down at the blanket. I had the sensation of being back on the elevator. The elevator I was so convinced was going up, that 2020—despite Covid—could still be my year. I felt myself free-falling, crashing down, yet again, to the ground floor.

"You need to see the oncologist, Dr. Reneau, as soon as possible, and we can get you started," he said.

And then he was gone.

And I sobbed. I cried and screamed long, excruciating wails. They exploded from my body and shook my frame. I didn't care who heard—I didn't care that Carmen was there. I couldn't believe I was back here—but not even. I wasn't back where I started, I was worse. I would have chemotherapy, which meant losing my hair and devastating my body. I would be weak, tired, and immunocompromised in the middle of a pandemic.

My biggest fear—the one everyone tells you not to worry about—had come true. The cancer was back. I couldn't deal. I couldn't deal at all and didn't want to. I cried until snot ran from both nostrils. I cried, hiccupping from lack of air. My mask was soaked with tears as I sobbed—I ripped it off my face. To worry about Covid right now seemed ridiculous.

Carmen placed a hand on my leg. She murmured platitudes about it being all right, and it would be fine. But I could tell she didn't expect this news either. No one did. My family didn't when I told them. My friends didn't either.

Cancer was like riding a carousel, a merry-go-round. Paris has many of them, beautiful ones, antique ones. Exquisite, gilded carousels, in front of the *la Tour Eiffel*, in front of the *Sacré-Coeur* Cathedral, and at the top of *Rue des Martyrs*, to name a few. As a child, I always liked riding the horses—the up-and-down motion made the ride more dynamic than riding in the chariots.

In July 2018, I paid the fare and rode the carousel. I was treated for cancer via a mastectomy and attempted to exit the ride. I was pulled back onto the carousel in February 2019—the cancer was still there all along, sneakily hiding until it was removed. Exhausted from riding the horse up and down—much like my life was going—I was ready to get off the carousel. See what other rides are out there. What else does the amusement park of life have to offer?

But here I was, back again. And this cancer was sneakier than the last, dodging the multiple tests, hiding within my body, ready to quietly take me out like an assassin. I was going around and around and around and part of me wondered if I had the strength to get through the ride one more time. Get through the ride for a second time. Get through the ride during Covid. Get through the ride without my family. I had no idea what was in store for me. I was terrified.

12

Illegitimi Non Carborundum

Going into my second diagnosis, my life was turned upside down. But one thing that my first bout with cancer had in common with the second was the foolishness that came out of other people's mouths.

Having cancer doesn't mean you want unsolicited advice, but somehow everyone believes you should be open to it. The things people say when you're diagnosed are wild. I can only imagine the things they think.

After all, you're the one in the "lower" position; you're the unhealthy one. You're obviously in a worse state than them, so why shouldn't you listen to them and welcome their help! And the so-called help—the well-meaning advice—can be anything from empty platitudes such as "Everything happens for a reason" to religious statements like "The Lord won't put more on you than you can bear" or my personal favorite, what is called "toxic positivity."

I was bashed over the head with toxic positivity the

minute I was diagnosed with cancer. Staying positive, keeping your morale and energy uplifted during a cancer battle, definitely has its benefits. It's easy to get depressed when you're scared, confused, and fighting for your life. But toxic positivity is a whole other can of worms.

Toxic positivity wormed its way into my life like an additional cancer. The minute anyone heard what I was going through, they admonished me to "stay positive and that's the only way you'll make it through." Gee, thank you, I didn't know my cancer cells would respond to happiness by completely vanishing.

In my first round with cancer, my elderly landlord had sat me down for a chat that I had no interest in. "You need to be positive. You complain too much about the apartment—about things that aren't real like leaks and bugs. If you're more positive, you can beat the cancer," he said. Of course, none of those things were fake—I even had pictures as proof. But as someone in a position of health, he placed the blame for my cancer on me and somehow believed that my mindset could change the genetic makeup of my body.

And he wasn't the only one who thought that way. Everyone wanted to place the blame on me as to why I was diagnosed with cancer. Whenever my family told someone about my health struggles, the common refrain was, "Well, you know, she does so much traveling—so maybe something over there gave it to her." Or "She's living in France, so who knows what they do there."

While I was recovering from my mastectomy in 2018, a close family friend posited I'd grown cancer in my body because I cut off a childhood friend. "Perhaps if you'd forgiven her and had a clean heart, you wouldn't have gotten this cancer," she said. Outraged, I screamed back the names of her friends and family who had passed from cancer. "Do you think *they* had an unclean heart too?" Harsh? Yes. But to say something like she had to someone recovering from cancer was insensitive at best, and cruel at worst.

Once, during Thanksgiving dinner at a friend's, someone told me I must have gotten cancer because the universe wanted to teach me a lesson. That I needed to learn something and that was the only possible reason why. She continued to attack me on this point, even when I tried to leave the conversation to save her from getting snapped at.

No, I did not give myself cancer. No, I am not to blame for the cancer cells that generated inside me. Cancer is a crapshoot, and statistics say three out of four people will have cancer in their lifetime. It just so happens that I had my turn early.

It was infuriating. I was going through one of the toughest times of my life and many people—knowingly and unknowingly—threw the blame back on me, while also telling me to be positive. Two things that directly contradict each other. And to say things like that dismissed the very real feelings I had—feelings of sadness and anger about why this had happened to me.

But the positivity actually has nothing to do with me. The positivity was for everyone around me. No one wanted to be around the crying cancerous woman. When people spoke to me, they covered their hearts with their hands, they tilted their heads, their eyes winced, and they took a singsong tone of voice, almost as if I were a baby or child. One friend burst into hysterical screams when I informed her of my diagnosis, so it was up to me to slap on a high-pitched voice and cheer her up. In addition to fighting cancer, I had to do the emotional heavy lifting.

No one wanted to be reminded of their own mortality by the possibility of my death at a young age. Placing blame on imaginary things I did or didn't do, places I've traveled, and feelings I had, helped others to pretend that the cancer boogeyman won't come for them. That there must be some way they can avoid it—if they can look at my life and not be like me—then the cancer boogeyman won't come. And I sincerely hope he doesn't. I don't wish it on anyone.

That's not to say there was no reason to be positive. There were many things to be positive about and grateful for. As crazy as it sounds, the timing of my cancer was both perfect and imperfect. The first time, I had just started my new job. I decided to stay in France and make it work—but at the same time, it was challenging. I often wondered if I made the right decision, especially when the cultural differences seemed too hard to bear. With this second diagnosis, the timing of a pandemic sucked, but I was glad to still be employed when so many weren't—and with better health coverage this time around.

I was grateful to be employed, but the lack of empathy while working full-time and having breast cancer was incredible.

I didn't love my job—it had just come at the right moment, and it allowed me to live in France. Plus, I met so many of my friends there. But producing videos and podcasts for a communications agency was not my passion—not by a long shot. I still longed to be in a more creative industry, one less stifled by office politics and archaic guidelines. The dream of international producing was still in the back of my mind, even though technically, I was doing it already, but on a much smaller scale.

Less than three months after my mastectomy in 2018, a close coworker, one of the few who knew about my diagnosis and surgery, pulled me to the side during a film shoot. "I don't know what's going on with you these days," she started, over a cup of coffee. "You're distracted and your work hasn't been great lately. I feel like you're not creative and on top of your game." I stared back at her, my eyes blinking rapidly in confusion. This coworker was not my boss—and I was stunned by the audacity of the accusation, especially as she knew what I had just been through. Her sister had breast cancer a few years earlier, so she knew how rocky the path could be.

You don't have a mastectomy and snap your fingers and everything goes back to normal. In shock, I mumbled apologies about being distracted and said I would be better at my job—and work as best as I could.

Later that night, anger burned in my belly like fire. Try going through breast cancer in a foreign country alone as a single woman and tell me how creative and assertive you're feeling at work. I sat at home, thinking of comebacks that would have been perfect at the moment—but it was too late, so I let it go.

When I scheduled my Valentine's Day reconstructive surgery in 2019, I sent the date of my medical leave to my manager to put into the schedule. I received an email back later that day. "Can you move this procedure to another date? It's during school holidays and people may be off skiing with their kids during that time," she had written.

Mind you, in France, school holidays are a very frequent occurrence. School-aged children have two weeks off of school every six weeks. In the workplace, parents tend to be prioritized for time off, despite the frequency of the school holidays, which makes it difficult for those of us who choose not to have or do not have children. By then, my boss knew I had undergone a mastectomy the prior summer. Either she wasn't thinking or didn't care—but infuriated, I knew I couldn't be silent this time. I fired off a snappy email about how no, I would not be able to postpone my cancer-related surgery so people can go skiing.

The lack of empathy astounded me. I didn't want pity—I hated pity—but a morsel of understanding would have helped. I began to wonder if it was cultural. I couldn't imagine people in America—at my old job—responding to me like that. They would be more understanding, kinder, gentler.

And sometimes, it seemed that people just couldn't help themselves. I noticed every time I told a man about my cancer diagnosis, it went like this:

"I'm a cancer survivor."

"Oh, wow. What kind of cancer?"

"Breast cancer," I'd say.

Immediately, almost like a reflex, the man's eyes would flicker down to my chest and then snap back up to my eyes. Never happened with women and happened nearly one hundred percent of the time with men. It didn't make me angry—it happened so quickly and so often that it annoyed me less and less. But it did still annoy me.

I started therapy after my first diagnosis in 2018, with an Australian psychologist so I could express my woes in my native language. And this lack of compassion was one of my biggest woes. I spent so much time crying in her office about my anger. Anger about my diagnosis, anger about people's crass comments, anger about not being extended grace in one of the darkest moments in my life. My heart ached for the US.

Is US healthcare outrageously expensive? Yes. Is healthcare a for-profit business? Yes. But I never missed American culture more. I knew for a fact that if I were at my last job, I would not have had these issues. I wouldn't be slapped in the face with a lack of consideration—either out of pure genuine concern or fear of human resources issues and litigation.

After my second diagnosis, my job informed me that they wouldn't fire me for the medical exam results, which was a relief. But they did inform me that the life insurance policy through my job wouldn't include cancer. I had to sign a contract stating that if I died from breast cancer, I accepted that none of my policy would be paid out. If I got hit by a bus, sure! Cancer, no. It was jarring.

I was starting to consider that maybe France wouldn't be the place for me in the long term.

◆ ◆ ◆

I STRUGGLED WITH TOXIC POSITIVITY and how to respond to others, but one of my biggest struggles involved my faith.

I grew up in a church-going family—every Sunday morning and Tuesday night, we were at church, for as long as I could remember. I attended a religious school growing up; all of my friends were simultaneously church and school friends. Once I moved out for college and then for life in NYC, I stopped going to church. I couldn't find one that I liked. But I kept up with praying and occasional Bible readings. I was still a "good girl."

I eventually found a church home in NYC: a young, hip, diverse church in Harlem that I loved. I loved and then left when I moved to Paris, where I wasn't inspired by any of the church options.

But I still kept the faith. I still tried to be the "good girl." So, if I was the good girl—if I kept the faith, tried to treat others well, stayed honest, and kept my heart pure—why did this happen to me? It was something I couldn't reconcile.

By linking my faith to my disease, I wasn't any better than others who blamed me for my cancer. I internalized that exact mindset but with a religious twist. That way of thinking didn't come out of the blue—I had heard those whispers all my life. After my diagnosis, whispers became shouts, as people sent me books by Christians with cancer, who seemed to have the same mindset. The authors railed against themselves and their lifestyles, and promoted the idea that if they had only been a bit more Christian, they wouldn't have found themselves in this predicament. They said my cancer was a manifestation of my life of sin. It didn't matter if you were a minister or a CME churchgoer (Christmas, Mother's Day, Easter)—it was all the same. Your sin brought this on you.

At the same time, I didn't think that suddenly going to church would heal me. I was religious, but I didn't ignore science. I didn't think praying until my knees were bloodied could spark a miracle. I didn't think my bloodwork would show no evidence of disease because I joined a church ministry.

But I did feel forgotten.

I left it to others to keep the faith because I couldn't any longer. People told me, "The Lord will never leave you nor forsake you." I smiled politely but, honestly, it seemed like he did both. The only faith I had left was faith in myself—the confidence I would try my best to handle whatever was thrown at me. I couldn't rely on the guy in the sky, because he let this happen to me not only once but twice.

I never told anyone how I felt. I knew my parents would be devastated. No use in upsetting them more than I already had. I kept it to myself—it was up to me to work out my crisis of faith.

It was hard enough pushing forward, keeping my head up, and putting a smile on my face with everything I was going through. I didn't need the onslaught of toxic positivity, empty platitudes, religious guilt, and apathetic or downright unkind people making matters worse.

There were two ways I could go with things. I could forgive those who wronged me, because life is short and I don't want any ill will. I could pretend they didn't say what they said or act how they acted, and greet them with false cheer every time.

Or, I could say goodbye to the negativity in my life—negativity that could have brought cancer into my life, not once but twice. I could say goodbye to those people and focus on myself, my health, and my ability to not just survive cancer but flourish after. I could create more boundaries to give myself the peace that I so deserved. I could give myself permission to be selfish at a time when I needed it the most. I think it's pretty easy to guess which path I chose.

"Illegitimi non carborundum" is a fake Latin phrase—popularized by the TV show *The Handmaid's Tale* (which is based on a novel by Margaret Atwood) but which originated during World War II. It's said that it started from the British army—but also from a US army general at the time. Since it's a phony saying, who really knows? But the meaning of this fake phrase stuck with me, especially since I felt beaten down by others around me.

I couldn't let the bastards grind me down.

13

The Frozen Five

I had seen the oncologist Dr. Reneau once before. Shortly after I received my first "all clear" from cancer, an angel had walked into my life. I was producing a video series at work about the gig-based economy, and one of my subjects turned out to be a gregarious private driver and tour guide named Sandra. Sandra was as kind as she was talkative, as excitable as she was warm. Her laughter erupted from her body like an explosion—it was contagious. She drew you in immediately. A Haitian American, she'd lived in Paris for over twenty years after growing up in NYC.

I spent the day filming and interviewing her around Paris, from dropping her son off at school to her afternoon coffee break and back home to spend the evening with her family. During an interview while perched on the hood of her car, Sandra explained that she had decided to make a major life change from being a nurse at the American Hospital to a tour guide after health challenges—she'd survived breast cancer. I shivered as she told her story. I didn't conduct her pre-interview, and the notes given to me didn't include anything about breast cancer. Goosebumps pimpled on my skin. After feeling alone for so long, I had met someone who could understand.

We cut filming, and I pulled her to the side and told her my story. Tears welled in my eyes as I relayed everything I'd been through, and all I was still going through. We embraced. I felt like I'd found a partner in the fight. We even had the same surgeon, Dr. Toussaint. "If you're still nervous, go see my oncologist, Dr. Reneau. He's great. He speaks perfect English. He can be a bit prickly, but he's great," she said.

And she was right—on all fronts.

I first went to see him after my second "all clear," in 2019, on the fourth-floor oncology ward of the American Hospital. Dr. Reneau was tall and imposing—a man who could suck all the air out of a room. He rarely smiled. He was intimidating, the exact opposite of his counterpart, Dr. Toussaint. To be fair, being an oncologist seems like a rewarding job at best and a depressing job at worst. I'm not sure there are too many oncologists who present like a ray of sunshine all the time (take that, toxic positivity!).

Oncology books were stacked high on the shelves of his wood-paneled office, the titles jumping out like a word cloud. Breasts, prostate, skin, lung: every type of cancer imaginable was represented on the bookshelf. I squirmed in my seat, the book spines in my face. A reminder of how bad things were—or how much worse they could get. There was no second-guessing what office you were in. I could at least find comfort that he took continuing education so seriously.

On the walls, in sharp contrast to the oncology books, were dramatic landscape photos. Photos of mountain ranges, rivers, and countrysides. "I took these myself," he said proudly. "They're incredible," I murmured. And they were. I appreciated a doctor with a hobby, and the photos gave me something else to focus on other than my health anxiety. If he was half as skilled as an oncologist as he was a photographer, I could trust him.

Dr. Reneau told me the same thing Dr. Toussaint had: they'd found the cancer was gone and I should go live my life. The doctors in the hospital met weekly to discuss their patients and findings, and to come to a conclusion as a united body and verify each other's work. "Don't spend your life in fear of it returning. If you have any questions or concerns," he said, sliding a business card across the desk toward me, "email or call me anytime."

And here I was again.

In July 2020, a few days after my second diagnosis, I found myself back at the American Hospital, back in Dr. Reneau's waiting room. It was different from the first time—mask-covered faces filled the waiting room—but the vibes were the same. Worry, concern, and anxiety. I folded and refolded my clammy hands in the pale-pink and white room. Much like my visit to the plastic surgeon's office, I was the youngest person in the waiting room and the only person of color. The average age seemed to be around fifty, sixteen years older than me. Patients sat whispering with their spouses, and adult children fretted over their parents.

This time, however, I wasn't alone—Sandra came with me.

Sandra provided an endless stream of chatter to distract me. I felt like the accused waiting for my executioner. Sure, I knew I would do chemo and radiation, but in all honesty, I didn't know what the details meant. I hadn't had much time for my mind to wander when I was called into Dr. Reneau's office.

"I'm sorry you're back here," he started. "So, we have to do twelve rounds of chemo, then radiation. You'll do two types of chemotherapy, four EC infusions—that's short for Epirubicin Cyclophosphamide—once a month. Then eight infusions of Taxol, a weekly chemo drug that is much easier on the body than the other one. We need to start as soon as possible." He flipped through his agenda. "It's end of July now—we can start in two weeks," he said.

"Hold on—two weeks?" I asked. Once again, everything was moving so fast—which was both a good thing and a bad thing. "Yes, we need to get you in chemo as soon as possible," he said. Sandra and I exchanged glances.

I cleared my throat and straightened my spine. Throughout this whole journey, I had felt like I was being dragged along without agency over my body, my health. I appreciated the speed with which my doctors wanted to treat me, but there was something important I wanted to do first. Something important I *needed* to do first: freeze my eggs.

I didn't know much about chemotherapy, but I'd read it

can cause infertility—whether temporary or permanent. At thirty-six, I knew my fertility was already naturally on the decline. Adding chemo on top of my age, I didn't want to jump headfirst into something that could end any dreams I had of starting a family. Permanently.

"Well, I understand that in France I'm allowed to freeze my eggs because the chemotherapy will destroy my fertility. So I'd like to do that first," I said. He flinched, his eyes narrowing behind his glasses. I wasn't used to speaking up to my doctors, especially in France, and especially one as intimidating as Dr. Reneau. "Chemotherapy doesn't always destroy fertility. And you need to start chemo," he said. "I'll start after I freeze the eggs. I insist," I countered. "It should only take a couple of weeks," Sandra chimed in, adding her support.

He began shuffling papers on his desk and leaned back. I could tell he was trying to suppress his frustration. But he relented. I would start chemo after the egg-freezing. I knew at my age, I needed to get this done—who knew if I would be able to have children naturally after putting my body through chemo? It was an insurance policy for me to plan for my future, even with such a big wrench thrown in my life plans. I didn't know if I wanted children at all, but I had to think ahead. Future Robin would thank me for this.

Chemo would start in September. But there was still one big problem—how can you find a doctor to freeze your eggs in August, in Paris? August was a dead month—everyone was on vacation in Greece, Spain, the French countryside, everywhere but here.

"*BONJOUR! JE VOUDRAIS PRENDRE UN rendez-vous pour cyto-preservation, s'il vous plaît. Oui, dans le mois d'Aôut. Ah oui? Bon, merci beaucoup.*"

I called hospital after hospital to get an appointment for egg-freezing, but it seemed impossible to find one in August. While everyone was off at the beach or in the countryside, I wanted someone—anyone—to freeze however many eggs I had left. Sandra helped, calling in every favor she could think of in the medical world, but I was losing hope. Egg preservation was not a widely offered practice in France, and most of the doctors were away for three weeks of vacation.

When Hospital Tenon, located on the eastern side of Paris in the 20th arrondissement, accepted my request for egg preservation, I cried tears of joy.

My oncologist explained the cancer this time was not DCIS like before—it was a different type of breast cancer, called estrogen-positive. Estrogen-positive cancer means estrogen hormones grow the cancer cells, which meant I would not be able to take all the hormone injections people normally do for egg preservation. I could still do the trigger shot—the shot that increases your egg size forty-eight hours before the retrieval—but that would be it. They explained that due to not being able to take the normal hormones, my number of eggs would be lower than that of most women, but at least I would have them on ice.

The process was intense. I took test after test—Covid tests, sonograms, and bloodwork—and signed piles of

French paperwork I could barely understand, holding the paperwork underneath the Google Translate app on my phone. Each time they asked if I had a partner and each time I explained that I'm going through this process alone and it's because I'm about to start chemotherapy. It was a depressing reminder each time. It didn't feel real.

The nurse, a young Black Frenchwoman, her hair pulled into an Afro puff atop her head, explained the egg-freezing process to me and the administrative side of having my eggs frozen in France.

"So, we will store the eggs and send you a letter about your eggs every year. And then once you turn forty-three, we will dispose of your eggs," she said. My mouth hung open in shock. "What do you mean?" I asked, alarmed. "France won't do anything with your eggs at the age of forty-three, so you can either pay to move them to a country that will do something with them, or we will get rid of them. We will send you a letter every year to remind you of the status of your eggs."

They asked multiple times if I was single because, at the time, it was illegal to do egg preservation in France as an unmarried woman. The only exception was for medical conditions or procedures (like chemo) that would affect your fertility.

France, as much as they tout themselves as a secular country, still had many Catholic-leaning laws then. Many women, including friends of mine, had traveled to Spain to freeze their eggs and start fertility treatment. My eggs would have to sit on ice in France unless I found a partner—

they wouldn't allow the use of donor sperm, IVF, or surrogacy for unmarried women.

Essentially, I needed to finish chemo, meet a man, and get married within seven years before my eggs would go down the trash chute. Not only that, but they would remind me every single year like, "Hey, girl! You still single? These eggs are waiting." It was jarring—the circumstances made me feel lonelier than ever. I was happy for the opportunity to save my fertility, but without the ability to use the eggs as a single woman, the pressure was immense. One major upside to balance things out, though, was that the cost of egg preservation in France was covered by insurance.

Later, in June 2021, the law was finally changed, after many years of protests (on both sides). Single women as well as LGBTQ persons can undergo IVF with donor sperm. Surrogacy is still illegal in France.

◆ ◆ ◆

EVEN WITH EVERYTHING GOING ON, I still made the time to date. My desire for companionship was stronger than ever, and no one can say I never put in an effort! It was exhausting—emotionally and physically—but also served as a good distraction from my drama.

This time, I met Jerôme, a finance executive. I liked him a lot: he was smart, had a good sense of humor, and was very easy on the eyes. He often showed up to our dates in a custom blue suit, fitted perfectly to his tall, dark frame.

He was from Senegal but had moved to Paris as a teenager. He came from a family of means—that was obvious—but he wasn't flashy or stuck-up. We spent most of our dates laughing at the silliest things or planning future adventures. He appeared to be the best man I'd met in a long time, and I was smitten. We felt good together and looked good together. The problem? He always claimed he was "so busy, I'm working so much" that we didn't see each other often. His lack of making time for me doomed the relationship to end.

There was a big shift in my mindset after my second diagnosis—or rather, during my egg preservation. Prior to the process, having children never ranked high for me, but I knew I wanted to get married. With the shocking news that they would destroy my frozen eggs at forty-three, something shifted in me at that moment. I viewed life differently—or more specifically, my love life.

No more dating for fun. No more Tinder roulette. I needed to date with a purpose, with a hard-and-fast deadline, to ensure my eggs wouldn't go to waste. A huge shift for a woman who never really thought much about having kids—just that it would either happen or it wouldn't. Now, it felt wrong to have the eggs there, frozen, without attempting to use them.

This was my mindset: *Time is running out*. My life clock could be running out due to cancer and my biological clock was running out as well. But with the egg-freezing and impending chemo, I put Jerôme out of my mind. I couldn't focus on someone who never made time to see me regularly, anyway.

Every few weeks, Jerôme continued to text to see how I was doing. Although we were dating when I had my biopsy, I didn't tell him about my possible cancer recurrence. Why open up to someone who never makes time for you? Despite my mania over time running out, I still didn't give him the time of day. I would either text a one-word response or not reply—after all, our last exchange left me miffed, and he was too busy for any type of relationship. After a while, I stopped hearing from him.

◆ ◆ ◆

THE EGG-PRESERVATION PROCESS WAS COMPLICATED, and I was still wrapping my head around having to do chemo. I couldn't clear my head with a trip to London—like I did before my mastectomy—because the borders were still closed thanks to Covid. I craved a trip there, to become anonymous in the double-decker buses and markets. But I needed to find another place where I could get away and process.

So I booked a quick trip to the South of France. I loved traveling within France—for a country the size of Texas, there are many different climates and topographies. In three hours you can go from snow to beach to mountains, and for a lower price than traveling from DC to NYC. Efficient, reasonably priced trains running multiple times a day made it easy. I had played in the snow in Chamonix, sampled the gastronomy in Lyon, tasted the wine in Bordeaux, and strolled the *Promenade des Anglais* in Nice.

This time, my travels in France would take me to Montpellier.

Stepping off the train in Montpellier, it felt like July 2018. Once again, I was on a trip where no one knew what I was going through—I didn't have the weight of my problems visible for everyone to see. I was just on holiday, like most of the country in August.

I enjoyed blush glasses of Provence rosé while overlooking the Lez River. I strolled the narrow streets, blocked on both sides by the cream-colored buildings of the South of France. I snapped photos of the street art—large, colorful murals, massive portraits of women with fierce gazes painted on the buildings. I sipped coffee on the grand plazas, people-watching behind my reflective sunglasses and jotting down the day's journal entry. I pushed my problems back to the far reaches of my mind.

While people-watching in Montpellier, I didn't have the joy I felt on my London trip, but I did feel at peace. It's a less busy city than Paris, and with the borders closed, tourism wasn't overwhelming. I trekked to Sète, renowned for its seven miles of beaches. I walked all seven miles of the beach, taking in the salty smell of the ocean and the cool breeze on my face. I paused to admire the docked boats in the city harbor, everything from speedboats to yachts.

I finished my trip with a stop in Aix-en-Provence, the famed landlocked town. I admired the pink buildings and learned about the town's history on *Le Petit Train*, taking the bumpy ride through the cobblestoned streets. I met up with a friend who had recently moved there and caught up on life over a long lunch with a bottle of rosé.

It was *une petite pause* from my real life, as the French would say. But my three-city tour was winding down and soon I'd be back in the world of tests, needles, and hospitals. On my last evening in Aix-en-Provence, I went to a pharmacy and filled the prescription for my trigger shot. Alone in my tiny hotel room, I plunged the needle into my stomach. In forty-eight hours, my egg-preservation journey would begin.

◆ ◆ ◆

THE EGG-PRESERVATION EXPERIENCE WAS A mélange of a comedy of errors and drama. I had recently made friends with the owner of a crystal shop in Montmartre. She was an American woman who had just moved to Paris, and I often stopped by her shop for tea or simply to chat. I wasn't a huge believer in crystals, but after everything I'd been through, I wasn't one to rule anything out, either. I had several friends who swore by placing crystals on their desks, nightstands, and anywhere special where good energy was needed. After several visits to the shop, I was gifted with a sachet of crystals to carry with me for my retrieval—to enhance my feminine energy and aid in my recovery. "Carry these with you when you need a little boost," she explained.

On my way to the hospital for the procedure, I pulled out the crystals to show Carmen—right at the exact moment the Uber hit a massive Parisian pothole. The crystals flew into the air. Into the air and perhaps deep into the filthy seat crevices of the cab. I mean, I don't really know, because despite cramming our fingers into and around the backseat, the crystals were never found. All I got were nails jammed with taxi seat crumbs.

We met Sandra at the hospital and headed straight for the billing department, per the instructions. As we approached the long row of plexiglass admin booths, my eye caught a sign taped up in several places around the room. In bold-lettered French, all caps, it read: IT IS ILLEGAL TO ATTACK AN EMPLOYEE OF THE HOSPITAL AND PUNISHABLE BY LAW. When you see a sign like that, it's basically a warning that you are about to deal with either 1) attitude or 2) incompetence. And in the worst of cases, both.

I dealt with the worst-case scenario. The bored woman behind the glass refused to admit me for my scheduled procedure unless I produced a *Carte Vitale*. She refused to understand I could still have my procedure without it, and that I was paying out of pocket and would be reimbursed by private insurance. She was particularly unmoved by my accented French and flowing tears over possibly missing the short window of time I had to preserve my eggs.

Sandra's unflappable charm worked in the end, and I was rushed to intake to get my eggs preserved. This hospital was not like the clinic where I'd had my previous surgeries—the orderlies and nurses were firm and no-fuss, likely because they were upset to have drawn the short stick to work during the most popular vacation time. It was also my first experience in a French public hospital, lying in a bare and austere room with a less-than-inspiring cold breakfast. At least I had a croissant.

As they pumped my arm with general anesthesia, the doctor announced to the room, "*On est prêt,*" telling the room I was ready. "I'm still awake," I screamed. The entire room laughed at my outburst, and I was assured by the anesthesiologist that he didn't mean we would start right that minute. I didn't know—and I was a bit on edge.

In the end, I went through two egg retrievals. The second went more smoothly than the first. The entire egg-freezing procedure was nerve-racking. I had to trust my body to do the best it could—produce as many eggs as possible—and there was nothing I could do to support the process. There was a total loss of control, which you would think I would be familiar with by now. But it was still disconcerting.

I ended up with five eggs—affectionately nicknamed "The Frozen Five." The number was disappointing, especially when so many of my friends have gone through the same process but are allowed to do hormone shots and lament the eight, ten, twelve, or twenty-five eggs they preserved.

"All you need is one," my friends said. Which is not true, but I appreciated the sentiment. The Frozen Five nickname helped—it gave them a superhero status, and made me think less about the likelihood of ever getting to use them, or if they would survive the unfreezing process, fertilization, genetic testing, and then implantation. All that mattered was that they survived in my body—currently an unforgiving environment—long enough to be preserved.

14

And So It Begins

With The Frozen Five sitting on ice, my chemo start date was fast approaching. I went through a litany of tests and procedures: a cardiology appointment to ensure my heart could handle the chemo drugs, several blood tests (which were always dramatic due to the difficulty of finding my veins), and an excruciating procedure under local anesthesia to place a catheter in my chest to receive the chemo infusions. I learned so much medical French in the process.

I whimpered, cried, and yelped as my neck and chest were sliced open and the chemo port was pushed into the opening. The nurse held my hand and wiped my tears. "You're almost done. Tell me about a book you read. Tell me about your family," she whispered in halting English, while dabbing my tears. I regretted turning down the option of general anesthesia, believing the story I was sold that the procedure was simple and fairly painless. Simple, maybe, but even with the local anesthesia, nothing can prepare you for having your chest sliced open and a medical device the size of a poker chip being planted inside.

Port in place, I now had yet another foreign object in my chest.

❖ ❖ ❖

I WAS PREPARING FOR THE next stage of my life: several months of treatment. I felt numb, going from appointment to appointment, while simultaneously managing the emotions of concerned friends and family. I didn't allow myself the time to think of what was coming next. I was facing uncharted territory.

"Do you want to have a party before chemo? Like one last hurrah?" I was hanging out with Carmen and her husband. I was at their apartment so often it felt like an extension of my own. Sometimes, I was even there without them. It was one of my safe spaces in Paris.

"We partied with my friend in the US before she started chemo, so maybe it would be a good morale boost for you," she said. The truth was, I was so overwhelmed with everything that I hadn't had fun in a long time. A very long time. My trip to the South of France was nice—but while it had been calming and relaxing, the drama that followed with egg-freezing and my port surgery had me stressed again. I needed to let loose, get crazy, release all the tension I held in my body. Tension that manifested in sleepless nights, an aching back and shoulders, and a consistently clenched jaw.

"Sure, let's do it," I decided. And do it, we did.

We started the night with a decadent dinner and bottle after bottle of wine. We blasted music until the wee hours of the morning, wildly dancing along to old-school music: everything from Luis Fonsi to Juvenile to Sean Paul. We recorded videos of our dancing and singing and sent them to friends in the US, doubling over with laughter at their reaction. I crashed on their couch, exhausted and happy, not worried about the foggy head I'd have in the morning. It was a good memory to hold on to when I faced what was ahead. A perfect night to end a far-from-perfect summer fraught with tears, confusion, pain, anxiety, and fear.

◆ ◆ ◆

OPENING MY EYES, I TURNED my head to the right, as I did every morning. Sunlight peeked through the curtains. It was a beautiful September day. I gazed out of the window at the lush green trees in my apartment courtyard—the autumnal color change hadn't yet started. September in Paris is always beautiful. The days are warm but not too hot, and the rain that will become a mainstay in the fall and winter is rare. From bed I loved looking out of my window at the trees, slightly swaying in the wind. I took a deep breath, admiring the view.

Today, September 10, was the day that I would start chemo.

I laid out one of my favorite dresses, a retro-styled striped spaghetti-strap dress. I had bought it from a boutique on Canal Saint-Martin on a warm day of being a *flâneuse* around the city. I paired it with a black see-through top (it was September but not summer weather, after all) and put on my faithful white Chucks. I didn't notice at the time, but it was the same dress I wore to see Serena win her match in 2018. Maybe part of me felt like it was a lucky dress—or maybe a foreshadowing of what was to come, considering how inspired I was by her self-advocacy.

I meticulously applied my makeup: concealer, eyeliner, eyeshadow, and filling in my perpetually sparse eyebrows. I released my bobbed hair from the previous night's pin curls. Yes, I was going to chemo. But I was also going to look good while doing it. There aren't many worse places to go in life, but I was determined to keep my spirits up through fashion.

It could be so easy to slip into a depression while going through this process. I had perpetually teetered on the edge of it ever since my first diagnosis two years earlier. I spent so much time since 2018 crying to my therapist about what my life had become, what I was going through, and the death of all my dreams.

Now, it was time to use every tool in my toolbox. As much as I hated the battle terminology, I needed to *fight*. Just like my London hair appointment before my mastectomy— I still believed that if I looked good, I could feel good. And I knew one thing for certain as I smiled and snapped a picture of myself in my full-length mirror: I looked and felt good. It would be the armor I so desperately needed. I looked like I had a hot date with a man instead of an IV full of drugs.

As my Uber sped down *Boulevard de Clichy* in Pigalle

toward the American Hospital, I slid my fingers over the smooth crystals—rose quartz, white and regular labradorite, howlite, and quartz. I had repurchased them after losing the gifted crystals, still holding hope for some healing power and good vibes. As I looked out of the window, this ride was a familiar one, but this time I was more nervous than ever. And for good reason.

The tall trees of Neuilly-sur-Seine didn't look welcoming—they looked ominous, their branches looming over the road. My chest still ached from the catheter placement three days earlier, and I was unable to take the nausea pill my oncologist prescribed for pre-chemo. I had issues swallowing pills all my life, and this one was massive. I placed it in my bag, next to my iPad, phone charger, and book.

"Carmen, what if I don't do this?" I asked. She had offered to accompany me to my first chemo session. "I mean, we can always tell the Uber driver to keep going and not go to the hospital," she replied. "Yeah, what if I don't go through with it? I could, right?" "You could. You don't *have* to do anything. If you don't want to do chemo, I'll support you," she said. "Maybe I could use the crystals—crystals and prayer could work, right?" I asked. I was grasping at straws out of fear. I didn't actually believe crystals and prayer alone could heal me. Carmen smiled at me sympathetically, but the skepticism was apparent in her eyes. "Bob Marley had cancer in his toe and never did chemo. He did die eventually, but he never did chemo," she responded.

"*Really*," I said incredulously. I mused on that fact, staring out of the window. "I feel like cancer in the toe would take a lot longer to kill you without chemo than cancer in the armpit without chemo," I responded.

It was a ridiculous conversation—I'm aware of that—but it was indicative of my mindset. I was going off into the unknown. There was no way of knowing how my body would react to the chemo. There was no way of knowing if the chemo would work. My mind went to my grandmother, who was diagnosed with lung cancer in her seventies. I remembered her living with us, coming home one night and projectile vomiting from a combination of her chemo and pain pills. She passed less than a year later, chemo port still in her chest.

I thought about Tiffany, my best friend's older sister, who I had grown up with. She battled breast cancer hard, multiple rounds of chemo ravaging her body. I visited her in the hospital in Philadelphia not too long before she passed. It was hard to reconcile the vibrant, hilarious, and creative woman I knew with the weak, chemo-bloated woman on the hospital bed. I didn't want to remember her that way. She succumbed to the disease at age twenty-eight.

What was it all for?

I could go through all of this, put my body through hell and back, and still find myself in a bad position—maybe even a worse position. I could do all of this, destroy my body, and still die in the end. Chemo is no joke. I had already put my body through a lot up to this point—did I feel strong enough physically, not to mention mentally and emotionally, to take this next step? Especially in a pandemic? I wasn't sure. My confidence in myself wavered.

When I first thought about The Paris Plan—way back in 2016—I had assumed moving to Paris and starting a new life abroad would be the hardest thing I'd ever do. I had no clue. This current battle would make anything else I'd done in life seem like child's play. Even the mastectomy.

Not having my family with me had me reeling as well. Seeing them on FaceTime wasn't the same as having them with me, as I had in 2018. My emotions were all over the place.

I rarely doubted myself. I knew I had mental fortitude, and I was smart. I was determined to be the hero in my life story, the main character of the novel. But the trauma of the past two years caused me to question my abilities for the first time. Was I strong enough? Was it even a question of strength, since many strong women—women stronger than me, like Tiffany—had died from this terrible disease? Maybe it all boiled down to luck. And maybe, this second time around, my luck had run out?

"You can always try chemo and then stop if it's too much for you," Carmen offered. I owed it to myself to at least give it a try. To do the most I possibly could to save my life. I would have to trust the process, no matter how scary. "I'll at least try it," I said.

◆ ◆ ◆

"I CAN'T SWALLOW PILLS; THIS one was too big," I explained to the nurse. She was a short Frenchwoman with a severe white bob. The severity of her haircut matched her mood as she stood with her hand on her hip in the chemo room. It was a bright, cream-colored room with a large picture window overlooking the garden. An oversized pink recliner rested in the middle with a long desk attached. I set up my crystals and iPad on the table, arranging a vibe for myself. A TV was mounted in the corner. Next to the chair was an IV stand—the only thing that identified the room as a chemotherapy treatment room. It hung with several bags and monitors, including one bag filled with a bright red liquid.

"Well, you have to take it," the nurse explained brusquely. "Can I cut it in half to take it?" I asked. "No. But you have to take it before we start."

If I had to take this pill before each session, one upside of chemo is that I'd become better at swallowing pills. "Okay, but please don't look at me, it makes it worse," I said. Carmen, seated in a folding chair opposite me, turned her head to the window to give me privacy. But the nurse? She stared sternly at me—like a prison nurse making sure I didn't cheek the pill—as I choked and gagged it down. It was ironic that an anti-nausea pill was making me nauseous on the way down.

With that out of the way, the nurse, accompanied by a more pleasant, smiling nurse, began to remove the bandage on my catheter scar, acquired only a couple of days earlier. "Will this hurt?" I asked. I'd asked earlier if I could put lidocaine on the scar to numb it, to which they said not for this first time. "It might be a bit uncomfortable," the smiling nurse replied, approaching me with an IV needle.

When a nurse says something will be "uncomfortable,"

don't believe it. When someone is stabbing you in the chest with an IV needle, it will *always* be more than uncomfortable.

She steadied me with one hand and plunged the needle through my chest with the other. The needle pinched as it went through the sore, stitched scar and then the catheter. I yelped with pain, but it was quick, thankfully. I exhaled in relief as she pressed to start the infusion.

"*Ah putain—ne marche pas,*" she murmured, noting the lack of flow through the needle. "I have to do it again," she said, as my eyes widened. Without giving me any time to mentally prepare, she removed the needle and slammed it back in.

My head swam as I saw white, then stars. The needle had smashed into my chest like a staple gun. Pain soared through me so quickly that my brain didn't have time to react. My body jumped in reflex, as if she'd used defibrillator paddles. By the time she started the infusion, my mouth hung open dully and my eyes welled with tears. If every chemo session was going to start in such a traumatic way, perhaps there was something to the idea of not completing all the sessions.

"Okay, great, that worked," she said cheerily, not noticing my immense pain. The infusions began—first, an infusion of Benadryl, to prevent allergic reactions. It also made me calmer, and sleepy. Then the infusion of the first drug, then the scary Kool-Aid red drug. The red drug, Epirubicin, is a derivative of the chemo drug nicknamed the "Red Devil" by cancer survivors everywhere. Epirubicin, like the Red Devil, is one of the strongest chemo drugs on the market and works by altering your DNA to interfere with the cancer cells. It's effective, which is good, but the name is well earned, as I found out later.

I was happy to have a private room for chemo—my experience with my grandmother (and television, of course) made me think I'd be in a large room, in a semicircle with other patients hooked to IVs. The idea of that frightened me. It wasn't that I was afraid of the lack of privacy, it was the idea that I'd grow close to the semicircle, my chemo buddies, who could possibly vanish one week at a time. The private room shielded me from that, as I only saw my fellow chemo patients through cracked doors when walking the hallway.

The rest of my first chemo was uneventful. After an hour and a half of infusion, I was unplugged from the machine and free to leave. A bit woozy but not yet nauseous, I tottered down to meet Sandra, who arrived at the hospital to pick me and Carmen up and take us home. It wasn't as terrible as I expected—I was happy to have one session down—but I was nervous about how my body would react to the chemo.

I didn't have to wait long to find out.

One hour after the treatment, back in my bright apartment in the 9th, I sat in my gray Ikea armchair. I had bought it just for chemo, the closest thing I'd own to a La-Z-Boy—a nice place to land after my infusions. Now nausea began to hit in waves: the room spun, and the television seemed to swing off the wall. My stomach roiled like the ocean in a tempest. The nausea was unlike anything I'd ever felt before.

I always prided myself on not getting motion sickness of any sort—a captain I met on a TV shoot once said I had incredible sea legs—but this nausea was ten times worse than what any normal motion sickness would feel like. I couldn't read my book, I couldn't look at TV, I couldn't look at my phone. The movement on television caused waves of nausea—everyone looked like they were moving on fast-forward.

My world pitched and I was dizzy. I didn't want to "break the seal" and vomit—I feared I wouldn't be able to stop. That was made easier since I didn't have an appetite at all. Carmen begged me to eat a lentil dish I'd made the night before—but looking at the lentils made me want to vomit. A glass Tupperware dish that made me salivate a few hours before now made me salivate differently. To this day, I cannot eat or look at green lentils. Just thinking about that dish turns my stomach.

All I could do was get in bed, lie down, and close my eyes. It was hard to believe I would have to go through this not one more time, or two more times, but eleven more times.

But it did get better.

By Saturday, the next day, I was able to eat applesauce, which would become a mainstay in my chemo diet. Anything apple became a lifesaver for me—apple juice, Granny Smith apples, applesauce—if it was an apple product, I could stomach it. A friend made bone broth for me—it wasn't available for purchase like in the US—and that became a great source of protein. Later my friends discovered that I could stomach boiled eggs, which became another diet mainstay. I drank copious amounts of tea—water tasted disgusting and metallic, a side effect of the chemo. I had bought a new fancy water bottle before chemo but now it was all a waste. I couldn't stand to drink even one glass of the stuff.

By Sunday, I ordered Chipotle for dinner—my first hearty meal after Friday's chemo. It became a routine for the next three months of chemo. Once a month, on Friday mornings, after choking down nausea pills (which did get easier), I headed to chemo. Sandra would pick me up afterward, and I would spend the rest of Friday and Saturday sick to my stomach, with masked friends in my apartment fretting over me as I wallowed in my nausea. By Sunday evening, I devoured my hearty meal of Chipotle. Monday mornings I was back at my "desk," teleworking like nothing had happened.

It sounds more simplistic than it was. The truth was the chemo ravaged my body. After my second session, I experienced intense constipation, so bad the neighborhood pharmacist hand-delivered meds my oncologist called in for me. I had to crawl to the front door, in immense pain, unable to walk.

During each chemo infusion, my sinuses lit on fire as if I'd accidentally inhaled a fistful of wasabi. It stayed that way the entire infusion. It was a side effect I wasn't prepared for, and my oncologist didn't seem to know much about it either. I started using a moisturizing nasal spray in hopes it would lessen the effect.

In addition to my sinuses reacting during the chemo infusion, I also had stomach cramping—yet another side effect that seemed to be rare. Thankfully, the cramping stopped once the infusion was over, unlike the burning sinuses. Chemo also made me freezing cold, due to the loss of red blood cells.

September 2020 was unseasonably warm—a slap in the face, since most Parisians couldn't fully enjoy it due to the Covid closures—but I spent most of my time indoors with the windows shut, under multiple blankets. Despite the ninety-five-degree weather, I couldn't get warm. I was freezing and always tired. The tiredness seemed to never go away with rest or sleep. I felt worn down in a way I never had before.

A few weeks after my first chemo session, I lay on the couch, under a blanket. My next session, my second one, was the following day, so I was resting in anticipation. My head was aching—my scalp was constantly sore for seemingly no reason at all. I went to scratch my scalp to alleviate the pain, and a tuft of hair pulled up from my scalp like a piece of carpet. It peeled off my scalp cleanly, like rolling up a rug from the floor.

I bolted upright on the sofa in shock. I knew I would lose my hair: the likelihood of keeping it during chemo was minuscule. I had even bought a few wigs in preparation for the day I'd go bald. But I thought my hair would just fall out—shedding that would intensify throughout the chemo sessions. I didn't expect it to pull up from my scalp, from the root, smoothly. There was a quarter-sized smooth spot where the hair had pulled up. No root, no fuzz, just completely bare skin, like nothing had ever been there.

I sat on the couch, staring at the balled-up tuft of hair in my hand. I brought my fingertips to the bald spot, rubbing it slowly, my heart thudding in my ears. I wasn't ready for this—is anyone ever ready? I had known it would happen but I wasn't prepared for the *how*.

I pulled my fingers back from my scalp, a renewed sense of determination swelling inside of me. Well, at this point, there's nothing to it but to do it. I walked over to my bathroom and cut the rest of my hair off. I hacked it off with scissors—ironically, the same scissors I had bought during the lockdown when I learned how to trim my ends. A lot of good that did me.

I hacked away at it, furiously cutting hunks of hair, then snipping more slowly as I cut closer to my scalp. The black trash bag on the floor of the bathroom filled with dark brown hair, and the sink with shorter clippings.

I stopped and stepped back to look in the bathroom mirror. It was a patchy job, some areas more closely cropped than others. I rubbed my hand over my (thankfully) perfectly symmetrical head. You never really know what it looks like under all that hair.

I knew what I was up against, what I was in the middle of, prior to losing my hair, but losing it made it feel more real. The saying "Thank God I don't look like what I've been through" is one I always liked, but it no longer applied to me. It was here. My hair was gone. I had a chink in my armor.

I went to a salon later in the week to have my head shaved clean. My eyebrows, as sparse as they were to begin with, soon followed. My eyelashes were the last to go, and despite tons of practice, I never figured out how to put fake eyelashes on.

The next day, I slapped on a wig, an off-the-shoulder sweater, and a leather skirt. I put a headband on as my lace-front wig skills weren't quite at the level I wanted them to be. I pulled on my tights and a pair of black, knee-length heeled boots. I headed off to chemo.

One down, eleven to go.

◆ ◆ ◆

I WAS MONITORED CLOSELY WHILE undergoing chemotherapy. I trudged up to the American Hospital two days before every chemo session to get my bloodwork done. Once a month, I offered up my wrist—my arm was impossible to draw blood from—for multiple vials. If I had enough white blood cells, I could proceed with the next chemo session.

After each blood draw, my oncologist, Dr. Reneau, discussed the blood test results and assessed how I was handling the chemo. "It's fine," I would say weakly. I had no choice—rather, I'd made my choice. Even though chemo was no guarantee, I wasn't setting out to be the new Bob Marley.

I grew weaker and weaker with each session—and my period was still coming like clockwork. Chemo normally stops a woman's period but, apparently, mine was too dedicated. Dr. Reneau prescribed Zoladex, an injection to suppress my ovaries, to protect them from the chemo and stop my period so I could keep more red blood cells. I went to the pharmacy and later plunged the needle into my belly while standing in my living room.

Those were the good visits—good bloodwork and chemo proceeding as normal. But it didn't always go this way. If I didn't have enough white blood cells to do the chemo, not only would it prolong my chemo schedule because that session would be canceled, but I would also have to get the "hell shot."

Neulasta, a.k.a. the hell shot, is an injection prescribed to help regenerate white blood cells. I don't fear needles—never have; I did my egg preservation and Zoladex injections on my own—but I feared this one. The pharmacy sent over a nurse, a Black Frenchwoman, to do this injection. She came into my apartment, looking around in surprise.

"Vous-êtes toute seule?"

"Oui, je suis Americaine. Je suis célibataire et ma famille habite aux Etats-Unis," I said, explaining that yes, I'm here all alone and my family is abroad. Her face clouded, and she gave me a pained glance.

The injection itself didn't hurt, but the side effects were terrible. After the injection in my stomach, my body felt like it was hit by a tractor trailer, and then dragged a few miles for good measure. My bones ached: it hurt to move, it hurt to sit, it hurt to lie down. So much pain, plus it prolonged my chemo schedule on top of it all.

I hated it here.

But oddly enough, the pandemic conditions were one

of the upsides of my situation. Unlike my first bout with cancer, I wasn't missing out on life, such as not being able to celebrate big events like the World Cup, or by not using my Beyoncé tickets. I was at home, in front of the TV, clapping at 7 p.m. and having Zoom happy hours, like the rest of the world. I didn't have to worry about job security or missing too many days at work, because no one was in the office anyway. The playing field was level.

The major downside of the Covid situation was the fear that came with it. I had a tight rotation of friends who would help me on my chemo weekends—Covid-cautious friends. Carmen started a MealTrain, a calendar where people could sign up to help me after my chemo sessions. Many friends wanted to visit me, but I didn't want to take the risk as an immunocompromised person. I had no idea what a Covid infection could mean for someone like me. Could Covid kill me? I didn't know and I didn't want to find out.

I received gifts from friends—soups, desserts, Bolognese sauce, and more—from the hallway of my building: me, masked, seated in my apartment doorway, and them, masked, on the stair landing. It was a true social distancing catch-up.

Some were allowed into the apartment but wore N95 masks and scrubbed in at the kitchen sink like surgeons doing open-heart surgery. One friend couldn't make her MealTrain scheduled time, so she sent her husband instead—we ate burgers and watched Netflix together.

People showed up for me in different ways, even from afar. Lauren, my cancer mentor, shipped a box of items to help me during chemo, including turbans that I wore often.

My family also sent me a box of goodies, some from them directly and some that I ordered myself and asked them to ship, including extra wigs and adult coloring books to lower my stress levels.

In Paris, some friends kept their distance entirely—they were too afraid to see me at all, knowing they would feel guilty if I fell ill after a visit.

By the end of October, it didn't matter anyway—France entered a second lockdown. But this lockdown was new and improved. The French government took into account the complaints from the first lockdown and now allowed people to exit their homes if they had a permission slip—a piece of paper explaining why they were leaving their homes. There were only a few acceptable reasons, such as going to work, walking a dog, shopping for groceries, seeing a doctor, and helping a sick friend.

The idea of the permission slip was wild: you were expected to be truthful and honorable in your reasoning. You signed it yourself, and you were not allowed to tap it out on your phone. It had to be handwritten on a piece of paper. It was a very French concept, as an *"attestation sur l'honneur"* is a common document in French bureaucracy. Later, they allowed digital permission slips.

Unlike the first lockdown, where I stayed indoors for two months, I had my regular appointments at the hospital, so I left home frequently. I never felt lonely because my friends were able to come over with the "sick friend" excuse on their permission slips.

While I wasn't lonely, going through everything without my family was still scary. Thank God for technology. After my second chemo session, the hospital rules changed as a new wave of Covid battered France. Cases spiked to almost thirty thousand a day—the highest rate in all of Europe. Just when I started to settle into my chemo routine, I wasn't allowed to have a friend accompany me anymore. Being completely alone during infusions would be a big adjustment.

My sister offered to be with me virtually—via FaceTime—during my chemo sessions, despite the six-hour time difference. I arrived at chemo in the morning—at 10 or even 9 a.m.—and would call her on FaceTime, propping her up against my water bottle. Even at 3 a.m. (her time), my sister would answer from her bed, chatting with me during the whole procedure. Sometimes Mila—her Maltese puppy and my dog-niece—wanted to be on camera too, not wanting to feel left out.

During one chemo session, we were surprised by a visitor. A nutritionist came to see me, a service offered by the hospital. She weighed me and explained what type of diet I should follow during treatment. I was thankful my sister was there to listen and to help me with details I may have missed or forgotten.

After that nutritionist visit, my mother began to feel left out. For a woman over seventy, she somehow has not rid herself of FOMO—Fear of Missing Out. My mother put herself on the chemo schedule with me. She is a night owl like me, and my sister is a morning person—so if the chemo was scheduled for 8 or 9 a.m. (2 or 3 a.m. East Coast time), she would take the call. Anything after 10 a.m. Paris time would be a call to my sister.

The chemo nurses couldn't believe it. At 8 a.m. France time, which was 2 a.m. in DC, my mother answered, much to their shock and awe. "That's your mom? It's the middle of the night there, right?" my favorite nurse, Anne-Victoire, would ask. "Hi, Mom! How are you doing?" she would say in her heavily accented English, my mom flushing, embarrassed to be seen in her bonnet and caftan.

I settled into a routine, albeit not a routine anyone would want to deal with. As my body bloated, my skin darkened, and fuzz appeared on my scalp like a baby duckling's, I started to feel like I could handle it. I could take all of the chemo on. I still struggled with nausea and sinus pain—and exhaustion and lack of appetite—but by now it was nothing I couldn't handle.

And then came the Taxol.

15

A Holiday Season Unlike Any Other

"This chemo drug is easier than the other one. That's why it's once a week. It's much lighter, and you shouldn't feel as tired or nauseous," Dr. Reneau explained. I sat slumped in his office, my bald head covered with a turban. While I still dressed up for chemo, the oncology appointments were a different story. Turbans and jeans were my uniform.

I finished my four rounds of EC chemo—I'm in the home stretch, I thought. "I take it every week—but do I get a break for Christmas?" I asked. "No, we have you scheduled for December twenty-sixth chemo."

A Christmas without my family? Away from home? I dropped my head. It would be my first time, and I was devastated. The borders were still closed to non-European residents. Now that I couldn't fly home, even for a brief period of time, my family had to see if an exception would be made for them to fly to me. After all, people had launched a "Love Has No Borders" campaign to be reunited with their

French boyfriends, so surely my parents could come to see their cancer-stricken daughter. Most of my local friends who could travel would be away at Christmas, and I wouldn't have anyone to help me after my chemo sessions.

We sent a letter to the French Ministry of Interior to request an exception. It came back with a semifavorable response. Yes, someone in my family could come, but only one person in my family could come—not the whole Swiss Family Robinson.

Deciding between my septuagenarian parents and my sister, who often acted as a caretaker for them, proved to be too difficult. If only my sister came, then my parents would be alone in the pandemic. If one of my parents came, they would risk getting Covid on the way over, a risk that could prove fatal at their age. There was also the overall risk of any of them getting Covid en route and bringing it to me in Paris.

In the end, I had to spend Christmas without my family, but at least I was in the care of friends—friends who were starting to become my Paris family.

Unlike the previous chemo treatment, my Taxol infusions were once a week. The drug was lighter. But staying well was still a full-time job.

Every week, on Tuesdays or Wednesdays, I trekked to the American Hospital to complete my bloodwork. The weekly blood draws took a toll on my veins. "We use this one all the time, but it's starting to slow down," the nurse said as my blood trickled from the small vein in my wrist into the tubes. "Am I in danger of the vein collapsing?" I asked. She affirmed with a nod, averting her eyes.

In addition to my weekly blood tests, I had a standing Thursday appointment with my oncologist. If my bloodwork showed my white blood cell count was too low, we'd cancel the appointment and I'd get a shot. I couldn't administer this one by myself, so a nurse would come to my apartment and give me the hell shot. If my bloodwork was fine, I'd meet with the oncologist on Thursday, and by Friday morning I'd be back in the chair to get my Taxol infusion. All the while, I feared getting Covid, changing out my masks as frequently as possible and aggressively washing my hands. I knew I was high risk, and going to the hospital three times a week during the peak of a Covid wave didn't seem like the best way to stay healthy.

I was exhausted—but the Taxol didn't make me as sick as the previous drugs. By Saturday morning, I was up and about, cleaning my apartment or going to the grocery store.

As the holidays approached, the lockdown was lifted in favor of *le couvre-feu*, the curfew. We could go out as we pleased, but we had to be back indoors by 9 p.m. In a way, the curfew was worse than the lockdown. Grocery stores and pharmacies were packed at lunchtime, everyone scurrying to get errands done before 9 p.m. Standing at my window at 8:30 p.m., I saw people rushing to get indoors, baguettes under their arms, children holding their hands.

Despite the curfew, the magic of the season persisted. Christmas trees decorated in gold and red popped up all over the city. Christmas markets were banned out of fear of superspreader events, but you could still find tiny stands of mulled wine, and the scent of cinnamon and *quatre épices* mixed with red wine drifted through the air.

I bought myself a tiny Christmas tree—my first real one—and placed it on my coffee table. The overwhelmingly strong fir scent made me nauseous, but it was nice to have some holiday cheer in my home.

I didn't drink while undergoing chemo, but I allowed myself a few cups of mulled wine. I had to celebrate the season as best as I could. Life wasn't quite normal, but it was becoming my new normal. Things weren't perfect, but they were manageable.

◆ ◆ ◆

GAZING OUTSIDE MY BEDROOM WINDOW in the morning, I no longer saw the lush green trees of the courtyard. The trees were bare, and mornings were dark. The chill of early winter set in. I stumbled out of bed to the shower, preparing to go do my bloodwork.

As I stepped into the hot shower, steam filling the bathroom, something felt different.

The water scalded as it hit my skin, though the water wasn't too hot. The burning came from within me. The shower drops felt like acid rain and I yelped in pain, cowering away from the water.

I staggered out of the shower, my skin raw and hot. I shivered, my limbs spasming in pain. I didn't know why this was happening. I lay in bed, pulling a cooling blanket over me and turning on my fan at full speed, in hopes the breeze would calm my skin.

I lay there shaking, crying, hyperventilating in pain for over twenty minutes until the feeling passed. The feeling of a million fire ants on my skin. The feeling of my body being ablaze.

I sat up and perched on the side of my bed, grasping the edge with both hands, taking deep breaths. What was *that* and why was it happening?

◆ ◆ ◆

IT WASN'T A ONETIME THING.

The more Taxol I received, the more the feeling hit. Some nights I lay in bed unable to sleep, itching, twitching all night long in pain. It was worst when I was hot, which was often, due to the ovarian suppression injections I received. My body's hormones mimicked menopause, and I underwent severe hot flashes. I underdressed for the weather, often wearing a light jacket in thirty-degree cold, just to make sure my internal temperature wouldn't rise and lead to a sleepless night of itching. I pleaded with my oncologist for help—this appeared to be yet another rare side effect. He prescribed two daily allergy medications to take along with the Zyrtec I already took.

I was still determined to celebrate Christmas and NYE, even without my family, even with these weird attacks. I slapped on my turban for all my outings—I had stopped wearing wigs because of my intense hot flashes. It was a common occurrence to go run errands in my wig and whip it off outside during a hot flash. Staring onlookers didn't faze me—the fact that I was sweating buckets did.

On Christmas Day, I traveled to Nancy's house in the suburbs—she had invited me to join her family's festivities. We became close after that fateful meal in Switzerland when she encouraged me to move abroad. I spent time with her family often, and she even visited me in the hospital after my mastectomy.

We pulled Christmas crackers, a Canadian and British tradition, for my first time ever. I won the prize and wore a pink papier-mâché crown atop my turbaned peach fuzz. I enjoyed a couple of glasses of champagne, my bloated face lit up in happiness.

After dinner, Nancy gifted me a soft, fuzzy Costco blanket, to keep me warm after chemo. The night ended with opening gifts on FaceTime with my family, my parents and sister on one end and me on the other. Thanks to online shopping, they had their gifts from me and were able to send gifts to me in Paris as well. Christmas wasn't the same, but it wasn't as bad as I feared it would be.

By New Year's Eve, I was content that the holiday season was coming to an end, but happy to be alive to see another one. I trekked up the hill to the *poissonnerie* in the 18th arrondissement, to bring a special treat to the NYE gathering I'd been invited to.

Seafood platters are the traditional food to eat on NYE in France: massive, heavy silver platters loaded up with ice and topped with various types of seafood, from shrimp to oysters to crab, all served cold. As a Maryland girl, I considered myself a crab connoisseur—it was my favorite type of seafood. I'd tried the crab in France—a wide, dark brown crab (when cooked) with black pincers, called *tourteau*—but it didn't compare to the Maryland crabs and snow crab legs I grew up on and missed dearly.

I noticed my neighborhood fishmonger had a selection of snow crab legs, the only place I'd seen in Paris offering them, and ordered three clusters—to the tune of a hundred and fifty euros. Crazy expensive, but when you think of how far the snow crab had to travel to be sold in Paris, it makes sense.

I collected my order and cooked my crab legs with butter and Old Bay (brought from one of my trips back home), the salty scents washing over me like a wave of homesickness. I made cocktail sauce—it's not sold in France—another Maryland staple for crabs, careful not to make it too spicy for the party. I baked a sock-it-to-me cake—a cake I made every Thanksgiving and Christmas back at home. If I couldn't be in Maryland, at least I could bring Maryland to Paris.

The party was a blast. It was a small gathering of five people: we couldn't have more due to Covid restrictions, but smaller was better anyway. They were all friends who stayed with me on my chemo days, so I already knew they were Covid-cautious. I could celebrate NYE without fear of contracting the virus. We planned to spend the night as the curfew was still in effect, so we arrived before 9 p.m. to avoid breaking the rules.

A full spread stretched along the dining table, including crab legs, seafood platters, and southern cuisine cooked by the host. We sat around the table laughing and eating, ready to bid adieu to undeniably the worst year of our lives. We watched David Guetta perform on TV in front of the Louvre—completely empty—for the NYE concert. We even drank a bottle of 2012 Cristal, my first time having the famous champagne, to celebrate the end of the heinous year. We had all survived when so many others hadn't.

The next day, we said our goodbyes after a breakfast of leftovers, and I headed back to my apartment. I didn't know that the day of joy I had, even fanning myself over glasses of champagne and whipping off my turban during the hot flashes, would be one of the last normal days I had for quite a while.

♦ ♦ ♦

NEW YEAR'S EVE AND NEW Year's Day were always special to me. I believed in making New Year's resolutions—but I also stuck to them. I hated the celebration aspect of the holiday—partying for NYE was always expensive and overhyped, crammed into someone's apartment with no one to kiss at midnight or wandering the streets looking for a party that wasn't charging an arm and a leg just to drink overpriced drinks in sparkly dresses. The celebration part of it wasn't my thing, but the concept behind it was.

I enjoyed feeling the restart of a new year. It was a chance to begin again, to correct the mistakes of the year gone by. I abided by the Southern NYE rules—my house was clean before entering a new year and I definitely never had any dirty laundry. But I'm also a bit superstitious. I believed that how I entered the new year, where I was at midnight, and the vibes on New Year's Day would affect how my year would go.

After a crappy 2020, I believed it even more. I needed something to hold on to. I scoffed at 2019 Robin, who had thought 2020 would be her year, so I was more cautious about my expectations. But could anything be worse than 2020? A year where I was trapped by the government in my apartment, as millions died, and I was diagnosed with cancer—for the second time? I didn't think so. I entered 2021 surrounded by the love of friends in a beautiful apartment overlooking the Seine with good food and good vibes.

But New Year's Day was something different. It was one of the worst days of my life.

I went home the next morning, preparing to binge Netflix and talk to my family. As I lay on the couch, the itch began. First, not an itch, but a tingle. I knew my tingles very well—I knew in under an hour or so I would be enveloped in the itching.

I hopped into the shower, blasting ice-cold water and hoping to calm my skin and abate the pain. But the pain worsened, spreading throughout my body so viciously I couldn't breathe. This itch wasn't like the other experiences—nothing calmed it; everything made it worse. I clambered over to the couch, clad in only a silk robe. Wearing any other material felt like an intense burning on my skin. My skin was burning. I was burning.

I screamed. I wailed. I sobbed.

I called my mother on FaceTime, to feel not so alone.

"Hi," she said, always sounding chipper to hear from me. Her face immediately crumpled when she saw my state. "I itch . . . so bad," I gasped.

And so she stayed on FaceTime with me. She stayed on FaceTime with me for hours. Hours while I cried, screamed, and hunched over in intense pain. My body trembled from pain. I was being raked over hot coals continuously. I ripped my silk robe off as the intense hot flashes flared up. Minutes later, I threw it back on because feeling the sofa on my skin was too itchy, too painful to bear. Feeling any fabric on my skin that wasn't soft like silk or satin increased my pain.

My mother, propped up via my iPad on the coffee table, stared with a furrowed brow, fluctuating between talking to keep me calm and praying over me. "I just want to throw myself out of the window," I said to her between sobbing gasps. "I just want to kill myself and make it end." She'd pray even harder.

Nothing eased the pain. I ran from the sofa to my balcony, standing outside in the thirty-degree weather in my silk robe. The cool air gave me momentary relief. I rotated ice packs and frozen vegetables on my arms and legs—anything to cool down my body. I lay on the couch, tears streaming down my eyes, ice packs all over my body. It was, without question, the worst pain I'd ever felt in my life.

Was the chemo worth it?

At my first diagnosis, and then the second time, all I heard was that I was so strong. "You're so strong," people cooed, not realizing the effect of their words. I'm not superhuman. It is a medical myth—gender bias—that women have a higher pain tolerance. It is medical racism to believe Black people have a higher pain tolerance. I am suffering but you don't see it. You can't see my pain—all you see is a "strong Black woman." You tell me I'm strong for fighting and don't realize how that discounts all the people who didn't make it. I am a woman and not a racehorse.

And at this point, I was wondering—is it really worth it?

As I'm crying on New Year's Day, all the good vibes from the night before are ruined and my body is in full-swing betrayal, is it really worth it? What is the chemo—this poison—doing to me?

16

"2 Legit 2 Quit"

After a drama-filled New Year's Day, I wasn't sure how much more I could take. I saw my doctor for my weekly appointment before chemo.

"Dr. Reneau, I'm still itching like crazy. It's awful, I can't do anything," I pleaded. I still had over a month of chemo to go. He agreed to increase my allergy medications from three a day to five, in hopes it would shut down the itching.

It didn't.

I didn't feel that my side effects were being taken seriously. When the itching first started, Sandra called Dr. Reneau, as I was in too much pain to talk. "Next time you have a problem, you should call me, not your friend," he scolded the next time I saw him.

It shouldn't matter if a friend called for me. If my husband or partner called for me, would the response have been the same? There's no way to know, but I doubted it. I'm alone in this country that's not my own, in an unprecedented pandemic, going through a serious cancer battle. Does it really matter who calls my doctor for me?

Throughout everything, I trusted not only the process but my doctors. But if they overlooked something, who could advocate for me but me? I wasn't getting the help I so desperately wanted, so I needed to take matters into my own hands.

I pulled my laptop onto my itchy lap and did a Google deep dive. I searched for everything I could find, reading everything from WebMD to Reddit to medical journals. After hours of reading up on chemo itching and allergies, the only reasonable theory was that I was allergic to an ingredient in Taxol, which is derived from trees, which sadly, I am allergy-test-certified allergic to. In an attempt to stop the itching, I needed to lower the histamine levels in my body—and try to lower them naturally, since the five allergy meds a day weren't doing enough to combat my weekly Taxol.

My research led me to the low-histamine diet—apparently food like tomatoes, spinach, nightshades (eggplants and the like) could raise the levels of histamine in your body and trigger allergic reactions. Including things such as seafood (which I had lots of on NYE), liquor and wine (also on NYE), leftover meat—a random addition. From that day forward, I pledged to follow a low-histamine diet so I could live without pain.

And so I did.

I survived on applesauce, baguettes, and butter. When I needed protein, I ordered empanadas from the shop around the corner, but only enough to eat in one sitting (no leftover meat, remember). Did the itching stop? Not entirely. I was miserable. But I wasn't screaming and sobbing in pain like I was on New Year's Day. When no one will give you the solutions, sometimes you have to try to find them yourself.

• • •

MID-JANUARY, I FOUND MYSELF IN Dr. Reneau's office again for my pre-chemo appointment. "How's the itching?" he asked. "I'm in torture. It's awful," I replied. I slouched in my chair like a petulant teenager. I scowled back at him.

It felt like a never-ending battle. As much as I enjoyed baguettes, surviving almost solely on them was taking a toll. I was still itchy but not all the time. My weight ballooned thanks to all the butter, baguettes, and empanadas. I was tired of eating the same thing all the time and still not feeling one hundred percent.

He sat back and closed his folder. "Do you want to stop? The point of chemo is not to ruin the quality of your life. You can stop if you want," he said.

My mind flashed back to the car ride with Carmen, pre-chemo. I never thought I'd be in this moment—I was so scared to start chemo, who would think I'd be so far along that my doctor would offer me an out.

I didn't know if I would be able to forgive myself if I stopped, if I took the out. I was depressed and exhausted. I hated every minute of this so-called easy chemo Taxol. I would rather go back to the other drugs and be nauseous than deal with the constant pain from Taxol. But that choice wasn't on the table—I could either quit chemo altogether or push through the last few weeks.

"No," I sighed. "I can keep going." This wasn't my first rodeo with cancer—I was living through a recurrence. I would never forgive myself if I didn't do everything I could, push my body to the limit, to fight this cancer and ensure there wasn't another recurrence.

There was no guarantee it would work—there are no guarantees in cancer—but I had to do everything I could. I didn't feel strong like everyone told me; I felt weak. But I was fighting for my life with every ounce of energy in me, with the hopes it would be worth it in the end.

The decision was made. I would do another chemo session the next day. I went home and looked at myself in the bathroom mirror. My face was bloated from the chemo and my scalp was finely covered in soft, downy hair. My complexion was darkened—not a rich ebony color but a dull, dark, and grayish shade like a corpse. Chemo had darkened my fingernails as well—black crept upward from the bottom of my nail beds. The weight gain due to my low-histamine diet was apparent on my face and elsewhere—I felt pudgy. I didn't have my eyebrows and eyelashes, and my makeup skills with both were pretty suspect. All the things cancer took from me—as well as my confidence. Trying to look beautiful for each chemo session was becoming more and more of a struggle.

If I was going to continue the fight, I needed motivation. I opened my bathroom drawer and pulled out a brown lipstick. I began drawing on the mirror.

I stepped back and admired my artwork. The phrase had popped up in my mind while I'd collapsed on the couch in pain and excruciatingly itchy. It was corny, but it was true.

"2 Legit 2 Quit."

• • •

FROM THEN ON, I TURNED chemo into a party. I had to keep my spirits up to make it through the homestretch. I was in the biggest fight of my life, the hardest thing I'd ever had to accomplish. Makeup and cute outfits weren't nearly enough.

I woke up on chemo days and put on a playlist that I made specifically for them, called "Chemo Countdown." I blasted the music in my apartment, dancing around and singing at the top of my lungs to "Alright" by Kendrick Lamar and "Survivor" by Destiny's Child, and always ended the playlist with "The Final Countdown" by Europe. I would stop to swallow my large anti-nausea pill. I needed to amp myself up for these final days of the battle. When my friends arrived at my apartment before chemo, they often joined in my dance party or watched in amusement.

One cold February morning, I woke up and put on an outfit I felt cute in—a brown top my best friend Lauren had bought me for Christmas and a pair of black pants. I oiled my head and put on a pair of gifted statement earrings. I smiled back at myself in the mirror, gazing up at the mantra I'd scrawled in lipstick. Today was the last day of chemo. I put a box of Ferrero Rocher chocolates for the nurses in my bag and walked out to my Uber.

In the US, there's a tradition of ringing a bell in the chemo center when you finish.

It's a triumphant way to mark the end of a long chemo treatment. The American Hospital didn't have a bell—I asked. But when the nurses unplugged me from the IV for the last time, my mother, on FaceTime, brought out a tiny bell and rang it as hard as she could for me.

I didn't think I could do it, but I made it. And I fought every step of the way. I finally felt like I was on my way to being a true breast cancer survivor.

17

In the Homestretch

With chemo behind me, I settled into another new normal. No more weekly doctor's appointments, fearfully heading into the hospital multiple times a week during Covid-19 waves and peaks.

We were in our third lockdown, again writing permission slips to go outside. This time, at least, we were allowed to write the permission slips on our phones and many restaurants began to serve takeout. The situation was improving, slowly.

The biggest change was the vaccine. Covid vaccines were available in France now—later than they were in the US—but the rollout was confusing. Only for people in certain neighborhoods, certain ages, sign up here but don't sign up there, you need a doctor's note, you don't need a doctor's note. It's available and it's not—make sure you get Pfizer but maybe if you're a woman get Moderna.

Pandemic confusion was commonplace—in addition to the news articles and Macron's state addresses, everyone relied on word of mouth. I attempted to navigate the vaccination system, determined to get some level of protection before I started the next phase of my treatment.

Finally, in a small community center in the 13th arrondissement of Paris, surrounded by elderly Parisians, I received my vaccine. It was less than a month after the end of chemo. "*Ça va?*" the nurse asked, putting a bandage on my arm as I wiped my tears. "*Oui, oui,*" I said.

It was a major moment, a turning point in the pandemic, but I didn't expect to feel so emotional. I had spent almost a year hiding out from friends and unable to see my family at all, and there was light at the end of the tunnel. The shot meant I no longer had to live in abject horror of my compromised immune system. The shot meant someday, hopefully someday soon, I'd be able to step out of Dulles Airport into the arms of my family. The shot meant everything.

I also had the silver lining of not having any vaccine side effects, due to my compromised immune system. Finally, cancer came in handy for something.

◆ ◆ ◆

THE NEXT STEP OF MY treatment, radiation, was scheduled to start a month after ending chemo. But before that, we would do one more PET scan to see if all my hypermetabolic areas had vanished. The PET scan would show if the chemo worked or if I was back at square one. Would I light up like a Christmas tree? We'd see.

I sat wringing my hands in the waiting room. I'd developed "scanxiety," a term I picked up from the Instagram account "The Cancer Patient," but a feeling I knew all too well. I was scared for days before my scan, worried I'd light up and find myself with a whole new treatment plan. It was the moment of truth.

"It's all fine," the doctor said, handing me my scan images and paperwork. "The chemo worked," he confirmed. I exhaled, my shoulders slumping in relief. My PET scan was completely normal, meaning all my tears, my pain, exhaustion—and the itching—had been worth it.

But that didn't stop me from lying awake at night wondering if it was really true. After all, my last PET scan didn't conclusively show I had cancer to begin with. Could I really trust the scan this time? That thought kept me awake many nights, tossing and turning in bed. At least I had radiation coming up: anything that wasn't killed via chemo would surely fry during radiation.

◆ ◆ ◆

I WORKED THROUGH MY TREATMENTS—ONLY taking off the necessary number of days, to the horror of most of my friends. "Take off more time. You know France gives you so much medical leave," they insisted. It was unusual to work through your chemo and surgeries in France. Even my doctors urged me not to. But everything in my life was so entwined—I had to do a good job and be a good employee to not lose my job and then lose my residency and then lose my health insurance. I saw no other option.

"We're not like the US, you know, we don't fire people for having cancer here," the HR lady said to me sympathetically. True or not, it would be a risk I wasn't willing to take. It was an even bigger risk during the pandemic, considering that if I were let go, it would be harder to find a job.

I didn't love my job—in fact, I considered it to be one of the biggest factors for my cancer recurrence. Despite my years of experience, awards, and accolades, my position wasn't well respected. I had the respect of some of my peers, but in a toxic work environment, my responsibilities were often given the shrift: no budget, no resources, oh maybe that random person we picked up off the street can share your job with you.

I often sat wide-eyed, nodding my head at my boss, who would proclaim that we had to fight for us to get our respect. I shared an office with a colleague who repeated almost weekly that "We have to put up a fight"—and it was for anything and everything: for respect, for resources, for me to get a one-year renewal of my contract. Every day at my job felt like a fight for the bare minimum.

By the time my cancer recurrence happened, crying at work and witnessing people being berated by the bosses was a common experience. But it wasn't only the bosses—it wasn't unusual to see people in a shouting match with their peers. I fell victim several times to the underhanded tactics of the ultra-ambitious. And I was stressed. I was so stressed. My therapist was making a small fortune off of me, and I'm certain God was tired of hearing about it in my prayers. And on top of my workplace stress, I had to fight a major health battle.

The silver lining of Covid was working from home. Working from home was calmer: no commuting on the Métro with my stomach tied in knots every morning. I did my job without all the additional interpersonal stressors and politics. I would wake up at 8 a.m., have my morning coffee, slap a turban over my peach-fuzzed scalp (or if I was feeling fancy, a wig), and draw on eyebrows so I could emote in Zoom meetings. I'd ease into my Ikea armchair with my laptop on my knees and start the workday.

And this day started like all the others, in my chair, turban secured, laptop on my knees. I'd just started to dig into the workday when my boss, a kindly Scotsman, asked if he could give me a call.

"How's it going? Is the treatment okay?"

"It's fine. I'm tired but it's fine. I start radiation soon," I replied. "Good. Be careful because there's a lot of Covid out there." My boss hired me, always believed in me, and often took on a fatherly tone when we spoke. I didn't mind him checking on me—I liked him and we had a good relationship.

"So, what's going on?" I asked. It wasn't unusual for him to call me to check in, but normally it was via Skype as opposed to calling on my cell phone. "Well," he exhaled. "I'm going to be leaving the company. I don't know what will happen with you, but I'll be moving on."

I widened my eyes, glad to not be on a video call. In an often unstable and toxic work environment, he was one of my bright spots. I enjoyed working with him. As people came and went on our team, he remained stable. Not to make it all about me—but at the time when I needed the most stability, he would be leaving?

He explained what would be next for him and how I would receive a call from our bosses later in the day. I listened, my silence punctuated with sniffles. It was obvious the choice to move on wasn't entirely his—the pain in his voice was palpable, and it broke my heart.

I dropped my head in my hands as we disconnected the call. Finishing chemo, good scan results, everything was starting to look up. With my main advocate leaving, though, I wondered if I needed to use my radiation time looking for a new job.

By the time I entered my meeting with my boss's manager, I didn't know what to expect. I put on one of my favorite turbans, a colorful one, and a nice pair of earrings. People reacted better to my cancer patient appearance if I made an effort. But also—how crazy to be concerned about people's opinion of my appearance in the first place, while fighting cancer. But I digress.

The image of Teresa, my boss's manager, flickered onto the Skype screen. "Hello! It's so nice to see you," she exclaimed, her voice ebullient with fake cheerfulness. Another thing I noticed: people liked to fake cheerfulness around me all of the time. Perhaps they thought I was a depressed cancer patient, and they needed to summon enough cheer for the two of us. I felt infantilized.

Two can play that game. "Hello!" I replied, a bright smile plastered on my face. We exchanged pleasantries and her lips hardened into a line, as to transition us to the real reason we were on the call. I rubbed my sweaty palms on my hidden sweatpants.

"So, as you know, your boss is leaving," she said. "Yes, I spoke with him earlier, I know." I felt a flush of heat creeping up from my toes. "We will put you on someone else's team for now—we're moving everyone in your team. But as for you—we don't know what the future holds," she said. A hot flash crept up my body, rising from my chest to my neck. "So, in terms of you, you produce our podcasts. Who knows what we'll do with that. Who knows if we'll continue to do the podcasts," she said.

My lips started trembling as my face flushed. The screen became a blur as tears began to well in my eyes. "What do you mean you don't know . . ." I interjected softly, trying to keep my voice steady. She was oblivious to what was happening on the other side of the Skype.

"We just don't know," she said nonchalantly, tossing her hand. "It's a difficult time and—" And I began to sob. And cry and cry and cry. Not only was I crying, but I was hot. I was so hot. The hot flash took over my body and I ripped my turban off, fuzz on display, desperate to cool off. I couldn't hold it in anymore—not the hot flash, not the tears. Through my blurry vision, I could see my boss's look of alarm on her face. She was caught off guard, assuming her nonchalant musings on my job security would be taken much better. She wasn't prepared for this, but who really is ever prepared to watch someone dramatically expose their bald head while sobbing on Skype?

"I'm so sorry, I'm going through a difficult time with my treatment and everything and you said you don't know about the podcasts, so am I going to lose my job? I'm sorry for crying, there's so much going on," I gasped, trying to stifle my sobs. She shook her head. "Don't worry, I'm so sorry. Don't worry," she said. She hurried off the call, mortified.

I sat in my armchair, dabbing the last of my tears. I pulled myself together—and then I laughed. Laughter erupted from my gut, rippling my body. Not only did I humiliate myself by crying "at work," but I also had dramatically ripped off my turban. I'm not sure she would ever be able to look me in the eye again.

The next day, I received an email from HR. The email explained my work contract would be extended by two years, the longest extension I'd ever received. If I had known before that this was all it took, maybe I would have cried in front of the bosses sooner.

◆ ◆ ◆

BACK IN NEUILLY-SUR-SEINE, THE LAND of clean, tree-lined streets and nannies of rich women pushing strollers. This time, I wasn't at the American Hospital but at the radiation center at the British Hospital. More than at the chemo ward of the American Hospital, I could see how far reaching cancer is. The radiation center was packed—not just that day but every day. It felt like an assembly line of people whose bodies had failed them in one way or another. Lots of women but many, many men—and everyone was around the age of fifty.

Before starting radiation, I met with my radiologist, yet another person added to my Avengers medical team of cancer fighters. He explained the whole process: I'd have eighteen sessions over four weeks. Every day, Monday through Friday. Radiation would only be a five-minute process. It would take me far longer to get to treatment than the radiation itself.

"With your type of skin, Black skin, you will be more likely to burn from radiation. You will burn," the radiologist stated firmly. "So, if we know that, is there anything I can do, anything I can put on my skin to prevent myself from burning?" I asked.

He shook his head sadly. "There's nothing you can do with your type of skin," he said. That was that.

Radiation gave me my first—and only—tattoos. With precision, they tattooed small dots on my torso and chest to ensure perfect alignment with the radiation machine.

I lay topless on my back in the radiation center as the radiology technicians—both male and female—adjusted me repeatedly. Lift here, slide there, slide down—all while holding on to two bars at a ninety-degree angle above my head. After they adjusted me, they ran out of the room to start the machine, to shield themselves from the radiation I took without protection.

The whole thing felt unnatural. Unnatural and humiliating. I was used to whipping off my top for doctors, but doing it in front of young, cute, male radiology techs was a different story. Radiation dehydrates your entire body, which causes exhaustion and, as I found out, can cause urinary tract infections. I developed a raging UTI after one week of radiation. But all in all, the grueling schedule of radiation was the worst part of it.

It was exhausting to trek to the hospital every day. Since Covid cases were still high, I taxied to the hospital—but when I could and felt up to it, I'd walk the one hour plus back to my apartment, grateful to be in the fresh air and masking up whenever someone ventured too close. Staying active was important to me, plus I had weight to lose from my baguette diet.

My favorite radiation days were when I had an all-female team. One tech in particular would always comment on how she loved my wig or turban of the day. When I draped my scarf around my bare chest and plodded toward the radiation room, I never knew who I would have the pleasure of undressing in front of that day. I would lie down on my back in the massive circular machine, and they'd adjust me several times and then leave the room to start the machine. I'd stare up at the blue General Electric logo on the machine each time—the only thing of interest to look at during the five-minute process.

One day, I finished radiation and went back to my

changing cabin to get dressed. I was rooting around topless, looking for my clothes, when the door swung open—an elderly man in a hospital gown stared back at me in disbelief.

"*Excusez-moi,*" I said, grasping to cover my chest. "*Oh oh oh pardon, excusez-moi, excusez-moi,*" he said, rushing to close the door. I sat down on the bench and laughed. He was more embarrassed by the situation than I was. By this time, half of Paris had seen me topless anyway.

When I showed up for radiation again the next day, a masked elderly man approached me. "*Excusez-moi,*" he started, sitting down next to me. "*C'était moi hier—*" "Oh, it was you! It's fine, it's fine," I blurted in English. "Ah! You're American? I speak English too," he said. It was the old man from yesterday, this time fully clothed. As we sat and chatted, I learned he was here, like many of the elderly men, for prostate cancer. He profusely apologized again, and we wished each other well in our treatments.

At regular intervals, I met with my radiologist to ensure my body was receiving the radiation well. He was impressed with my progress. "Your skin is taking the radiation very well—you're not burning. What are you doing?" he asked. "After radiation, before I put my clothes on, I'm putting pure aloe vera and Aquaphor on my skin," I replied. "Well, keep doing that," he said.

It was incredulous to me that as a radiologist, he knew melanated skin burns from radiation but offered no solutions. He had told me I had no option but to burn. I researched on my own, though, and through a Black breast cancer survivor Facebook group, I discovered the aloe vera and Aquaphor trick. It made no sense to go through unnecessary pain, even if I had to find the solution on my own.

But even more important, why was a medical professional not well-versed in preventing the pain of their patients—all their patients, of all skin types? It unnerved me. It was a callback to my situation with the plastic surgeon. Despite knowing how badly I would scar, he decided to operate on me the same way he would with any of the rest of his patients—even against my own wishes.

❖ ❖ ❖

ALTHOUGH I WAS DEALING WITH radiation and on a dating break, I still yearned for a partner. My cancer journey made me hyperaware of my need for partnership. I was never a hopeless romantic—I've always been pragmatic about relationships and the type of guys I wanted in my life. In part, it's thanks to watching my parents' relationship while growing up.

Bob and Jackie met at church and married at the ages of twenty and twenty-one—and even after over fifty-five years of marriage, enjoy each other's company. Not only are they still completely obsessed with each other, but they have worked together, side by side, for the past forty plus years. They're such a model couple that they were interviewed about their love on *Today*—thanks to me submitting them to a colleague for a Valentine's Day special, one of my proudest and most embarrassing moments.

My parents spoke with *Today* host Meredith Vieira,

and my boss and colleagues gathered around my cubicle to watch. "You guys have been married thirty-nine years and you work together. How does that work out?" asked Meredith.

My mother, nearly unrecognizable in her studio makeup, replied, "Well, sometimes he fires me and sometimes I quit. It only lasts for about an hour or two. But I tell you one thing about working together—it's the one problem—is the sexual harassment. I get a little kiss there, a little hug here, a little peck there, and I tell him I'm going to report him to HR," she said, and laughed. And so did my bosses and coworkers, while I shrunk in my chair, mortified.

But you see what kind of family I grew up in, what kind of parents I was raised by. The bar was set high for relationships from day one. Breast cancer reframed my mindset and outlook on dating, though, particularly my desire for partnership.

Going to doctor's appointments alone and being a burden on my friends and family is not what I wanted for the rest of my life. They never said I was a burden, but I felt like one. Always needing help, always needing someone to stay with me—during surgeries, chemo, and doctor's appointments.

Sitting in the waiting room of the surgery and oncology departments, I was often the only person there alone. Everyone was there with a spouse, rubbing their hand and calming them before their big appointment. I saw people that weren't quitting on their loved ones—even in the darkest moments.

I appreciated my family flying to be with me for my surgeries for my first bout with cancer, but now, in the second bout, I felt even more alone. Even worse, being the type of breast cancer patient I was, I never saw myself anywhere else. I sought out breast cancer forums and Facebook groups. The image I saw staring back at me was not a reflection of me and my struggle. I knew Black women with breast cancer. I knew single women with breast cancer. But it was always the exception and not the norm.

Going to these breast cancer forums, hopeful, eager to read posts from women who understand what I'm going through, rarely yielded the results I wanted. Often, they were older and married, posting about how their DH ("dear husband," for those not well-versed in online speak) was supporting them through it all.

Breast cancer is growing among women under forty, and as women are marrying later, not only do we have to navigate it alone, but we also have to navigate dating after surviving a disease that cuts to the core of the superficial and sexist standards of dating in the twenty-first century.

What was there for me? What exists for the under-forty, single Black woman going through this alone? My experiences over time extinguished my hope that I would make it through to the other side and ever find partnership.

◆ ◆ ◆

A FEW WEEKS INTO RADIATION, Jerôme, the perpetually busy finance guy, popped back into my life. He never stopped reaching out—a "hey" here and there, an occasional "*coucou.*"

This time, he reached out and told me he'd lost his mother to Covid—and I'd been on his mind and he wanted to know if we could meet up.

I do not give second chances. As Miranda on *Sex and the City* said, "We didn't work out—you need to not exist." But again, something had shifted in me the summer before. My eggs were sitting in the 20th arrondissement waiting for me, counting down the years. Maybe I was too harsh? Maybe I should give him a second chance?

My bigger concern was showing up considerably larger and bald-headed from chemo. You can't show up looking completely different and expect someone not to notice.

Dating with breast cancer gave me anxiety—wondering if I should tell him, and when, if I did, was it too early or too late. After my first bout, my general thought process was to tell people in the beginning, to weed out the ones who couldn't handle it.

I'll never forget what Hoda Kotb, fellow breast cancer survivor and former colleague, told me in the summer of 2018 after my mastectomy, my face wet with tears during a heart-to-heart in her NBC dressing room. "Dating after breast cancer automatically gives you a higher caliber of man. You don't have to deal with the immature ones anymore, because your story will weed them out." It was something I took to heart and held on to.

So it was time to see if Jerôme was that kind of man. I told him ahead of time. "Before we meet up, I want to tell you first about something I've been going through the last few months," I started. "I didn't want to meet up and you didn't know." I explained my cancer recurrence and the treatment I underwent, sticking to the basics. I told him I look a bit different from how he remembers me, due to the treatment. To which he replied, "I'm sure you look good and pretty." Be still, my shallow heart.

I arrived at the coffee shop feeling insecure and anxious. I had put on a new skirt, painted my blackened nails, and styled my closely cropped curls. He arrived in a tailored blue suit, the uniform of French men in finance. And he looked amazing, which made me both happy and annoyed.

Over hot coffee on a cold bench, we discussed where things went wrong with us—a mix of bad communication and misunderstandings. I left the coffee date feeling good—I'd liked him so much when we originally dated, perhaps I was wrong to cut him loose after all. "I'm sorry I wasn't there for you when you went through chemo," he said, looking down at his hands. "I wish I had known. But I'm here for you now, if you need to go to a doctor's appointment or anything."

My second cancer journey greatly changed me. He seemed different as well, still grieving the loss of a parent but also more thoughtful. Maybe under the most terrible of circumstances, we both had changed for the better.

We picked up where we left off, going for long walks in *Parc Martin Luther King* in the 17th arrondissement, gazing at the cherry blossoms. Going for dinners and Sunday lunches, laughing and animatedly talking the whole time. People stopped us on the street to say how good we looked together. He told me that he told his father about me and we discussed taking trips together—maybe even going to a friend's wedding with me. It was just . . . easy. Finally.

In the end, he only paid lip service. The same problems cropped up. "I'm so busy. I want to spend time with you, but I'm so busy." Jerôme was so "busy" to the point that we would go over a month without seeing each other. All the while, he was still expressing to me how much he wished he could have been my caretaker during chemo.

Eventually, things ended much like the first time. I regretted letting him back in to give him a chance, only to have him hurt me in a worse way. Even more, I regretted that I made time for him during my cancer treatment, and he couldn't do the bare minimum for me. This hurt more than the first time, because I had wanted to believe him—and I unconsciously pinned all my hopes and dreams for a "normal" future on him. And ultimately, even my sense of self-worth.

As a child, I would spend my afternoons at my Grandma Jessie's house. Grandma Jessie was a tough woman, born on a sharecropper farm in South Carolina and moving to DC as a teenager for a better life.

She met and married my grandfather Ben, several years her senior but with the playfulness of a child. His playfulness was the perfect match to her seriousness. She helped raise her younger siblings, moving them to DC to live in her rowhouse. Her house was packed to the gills with random animals my grandfather would bring home as pets, as well as family members, including my mother, an only child.

I never knew my Grandpa Ben: he was murdered during

a workplace robbery, shot dead by a teenager, three years before I was born. One afternoon, over banana pudding in Grandma Jessie's narrow kitchen, I asked her a question. "Grandma, why aren't you married? Why haven't you remarried?" Grandma didn't even look up from the sink, where she was preparing dinner. "I can do bad all by myself," she replied with a sniff.

Grandma Jessie never remarried, spending twenty-two years as a widow. I didn't fully understand what she meant that day, and she definitely wasn't offering any explanations. It's something that's stuck with me through the years that I completely understand now. That's not to say I don't desire companionship—I do—but it has to be the right kind of companionship. It's not worth being in a relationship if you're still going through the hard parts alone. And sometimes finding the right partner, particularly in a completely different culture, requires kissing more frogs than you expect.

◆ ◆ ◆

I FINISHED EIGHTEEN ROUNDS OF radiation with minimal burns, thanks to the research I did on my own: only a tiny burn near my collarbone, an area that I didn't realize was being radiated, thus I never applied anything there. If I didn't speak up for myself or advocate for myself, no one would. I couldn't always rely on my doctors to find the solution for me. I couldn't rest on my laurels. I had to stand up for myself and find solutions for myself even when I didn't feel like it. Even when the very idea of it exhausted me.

Finishing active treatment was a relief, but mostly scary. No longer would I have the weekly doctor check-ins or the multiple blood tests in one month. If something slipped through the cracks—if an errant cancer cell still remained, lurking somewhere in my body—we wouldn't be able to tell until later.

Oncology is a science, but it's a science that's still being learned. After my first diagnosis, I did genetic testing to find out if I had the BRCA 1 or BRCA 2 cancer-causing genes. The geneticist explained, "These are the genes we know that cause breast cancer. You don't have them. But there may be other genes we don't know about yet because we're still learning."

Cancer is a sneaky disease. I knew that from my second diagnosis, which had evaded the blood test, biopsy, and PET scan. When you finish a successful cancer treatment, they say you are "NED"—No Evidence of Disease. It's tricky wording: it doesn't mean you don't still have cancer; it means they have no signs you still have it. There's no way to tell one hundred percent that the treatment worked. In the end, you have to trust the science, trust your doctors, and trust in whatever higher belief you have (JC for me)—or you'll drive yourself insane.

18

Life Is Short and Long

After one surgery, twelve rounds of chemo, and eighteen rounds of radiation, I was again declared NED—No Evidence of Disease. The next step was tamoxifen, an estrogen-blocking medication I would have to take for the next five years. The hope was, if used correctly, the pill would suppress the cancer-growing hormones, and I wouldn't have a recurrence. My type of breast cancer wasn't compatible with immunotherapy or other medications—tamoxifen was it.

"I read about all these side effects of the drug, including other cancers," I said when I met with my oncologist, Dr. Reneau, before starting the drug. "All medicines have side effects," he said with a shrug.

I wasn't forced to take it, but he strongly advised that I do it. I held on to the prescription for a few days. Then I held on to the box of pills for a few days, staring at them unopened on my desk. I remembered when I was offered an "out" to stop chemo—could I be okay with knowing that I didn't do everything they recommended to prevent having cancer again?

In the end, I decided to take the tamoxifen. Even with all the side effects—fatigue, hot flashes, pelvic pain, body aches—it was better than the risks associated with not taking it.

NED didn't mean all of my problems were over: I was yet again being forced out of another apartment. My dream apartment. The apartment I lived in while being rediagnosed with cancer. The one I returned to after chemo sessions. The open kitchen where my friends cooked nutritious meals for me after chemo and watched *Emily in Paris* on my couch while I napped away my nausea. I loved the apartment for everything it was before my diagnosis, and my love for it grew during my cancer battle.

Having a calm, beautiful oasis to call my home had greatly aided me in my recovery. It lowered my stress levels so I could focus on one thing and one thing only: beating cancer. I'm not sure how things would have turned out if I had had to go through the same thing in, God forbid, my Disneyland mouse-house apartment. I'm glad I never had to find out.

Shortly after my NED, the owners reached out and said they'd like the apartment back by June. They had no recollection of telling me anything about 2023. They said they were retiring and planned to live in the apartment. I later found the apartment listed online for six hundred euros more a month. The borders were now open again, and they didn't want it for themselves—they wanted to kick me out to charge higher rent.

I couldn't catch a break. Frustrated, I went to ADIL, the tenant legal aid service based in my neighborhood municipal building. "What he's doing is very illegal," the woman explained, after I showed her my lease and printouts of the online ad for my apartment. "You could take him to court and win, but it could take a while."

It was good to hear that I'd win, but I knew I'd never take him to court. I was exhausted. Mind, body, and soul. Everything I had in me, I had used to fight against breast cancer. The idea of entering another fight, even one I was guaranteed to win, felt insurmountable. Not only did I not have the energy, but also I didn't want to have the bad energy of being in an apartment where I wasn't wanted.

I had to let it go.

On the hunt again, I found a place five streets over. I wasn't ready to leave my beloved 9th arrondissement. But the quality of the apartment didn't match the great location. It turned out to be a complete disaster.

The apartment seemed dusty no matter how often I vacuumed, even with a professional cleaner. The furniture was broken—my bed had to be sat on in a particular way so the frame wouldn't fall down. And, of course, the landlord refused to fix any of it. I had had to find a place on short notice and it showed.

Shortly after moving in, I became ill—congestion, coughing, and sneezing for weeks. I took multiple Covid tests and cold and allergy pills, but nothing seemed to fix it. In addition to being ill, when I opened my windows at night, my place sometimes had a weird smoky smell. I was at a loss—until one day, walking around the corner to wait for the bus, I noticed something disturbing. I glanced up at the building next to mine, a stone edifice with a tiny plaque: "*Crematorium de Paris.*" My body involuntarily shuddered—there was no mistaking what the building was. I was living next to a crematorium.

All at once, my constant congestion and coughing made sense. As well did the random smoke and chemicals I smelled from time to time. I purchased an air-quality monitor and it verified my suspicions. The air quality in the apartment was horrific, at carcinogenic levels, every single day. I wanted to get out of that apartment—I needed to. I tried not to think about what levels of ash and chemicals I'd already inhaled.

I don't know if the God of Apartments had it out for me, but nothing could beat this story. I had to laugh—and buy an air purifier. And when I found a used condom stuffed in the crevices of the sofa cushions, I knew I had to get the hell out of there.

And I did, eventually.

◆ ◆ ◆

I'M HAPPY I'M ALIVE, I'M happy I'm alive, I'm happy I'm alive. I repeated this morbid little mantra, looking into my bathroom mirror. Maybe if I repeated it enough, it would ring true. I wasn't *unhappy* to be alive. My emotions were running wild—I didn't know how to feel.

Gazing in the mirror, I also saw inspirational quotes written on pink Post-it notes—quotes from famous Black women. "If you don't like something, change it. If you can't change it, change your attitude," Maya Angelou tells me. "It's not the load that breaks you down, it's the way you carry it," advises Lena Horne. I put those notes up when things got bad at my job and carried them to each apartment, strung together with silver washi tape. But the wisdom was for more than my work life—I needed it for my personal struggles as well. I drew my strength from these wise women during my hardest days.

The dark days arrived. When I was fighting for my life, there was no time to think about what's next and what's going on. Especially when things move fast. I saw so many doctors who were concerned about my physical health, but my emotional health was just as important. And I was floundering.

The feelings that set in after—the guilt. I'm happy to be a cancer survivor. I'm proud. But there's also survivor's guilt for being one of the ones who made it. Why me? Why not the others? Like Tiffany, like Jeremy from my cancer support group. It has nothing to do with me valiantly fighting—they did too. My survival doesn't make me any stronger than the ones that did not. To say so is to disrespect their memory and their battle.

I also hated the word "lucky." I didn't get lucky—what I went through was exhausting and strenuous. It wasn't easy.

Why did the treatment work for me and not for so many others? The guilt I felt after my first breast cancer journey was nothing compared to this time. I felt like an imposter then—now I felt shame for surviving when others didn't. Should I even celebrate my NED?

The post-traumatic stress disorder is something you're not warned about. My stomach hurts before doctor's appointments. My palms are sweaty when I'm getting tests done. I'm anxious several days in advance, plagued by a consistent sense of dread. Every summer, I fall into a depression—my subconscious remembers the trauma of the summers of 2018 and 2020. Sometimes I'll see something that reminds me of my time in treatment, and nausea immediately rolls over me. I still can't eat green lentils—the thought of them turns my stomach. I haven't touched an empanada since either.

Every single oddity in my body—a random pain, a bump here or there—increases my anxiety. Is it coming back? Or is it a new cancer, brought on by the hormone therapy I'm taking to prevent breast cancer but that can cause other cancers? I try to toe the line between not being a hypochondriac and staying vigilant on my health. After all, late at night, I still lie awake and wonder, *Is there anything I could have done to prevent this?* Had I gone to the doctor sooner, would none of this have happened? If I'd kept my follow-up oncology appointment in early 2020, instead of postponing it for weeks, would I not have had to go through chemo?

It's another form of guilt—the guilt that I'm not doing enough. Should I be vegan? Should I never eat a morsel of sugar ever again, even if it's in fruit? Never taste the sweet elixir of champagne when I'm celebrating a win in life? Can I even fully enjoy life ever again, or will the dark cloud always loom in the background?

Worst of all is the grief.

The morning of my mastectomy, when I took pictures of my breasts, I wanted one last chance to say goodbye to the girls who were with me most of my life. It wasn't only about the aesthetics—I mean, I adored my boobs. It was about so much more than that. With having a single mastectomy, I felt I was giving up my ability to breastfeed a future child of mine. I was giving up my femininity. I would forever feel not whole, that a piece of me was missing.

With the second cancer battle, I lost so much more than the first time. I lost my hair, my independence, and even my sense of self. And if I had missed the signs something was off with my health, could I really have confidence in myself anymore? My experiences in Paris (my job, the apartments, dating) had withered my confidence, and cancer destroyed what was left of it.

I froze my eggs but my doctors weren't confident I'd ever be able to have children. Whenever I mentioned future children, I was met with a sad smile. I could feel pity emanating from them. They wanted me to wait until after hormone therapy, and by then I could be too old—and who knows if the eggs would survive the process anyway. There was also a huge risk if I became pregnant naturally: with a history of hormone-induced cancer, I could be facing cancer a third time. I lost what I originally thought my future could be.

I had nine surgical procedures in five years, including

one to remove a tube of plastic from my chest that the surgeon who removed my chemo port left behind. My body was riddled with scars and keloids, and my days riddled with pain.

My chest disgusted me, especially the natural breast that was surgically botched. And it wasn't just me. Even Dr. Boucher, my gynecologist who declared years earlier that my reconstructed breast looked good, had to admit upon seeing the botched natural breast, "Oh, well, yes, that doesn't look so nice."

I rarely looked at my body in the mirror. When I did look, all I saw was a woman who'd lost so much.

As my friends all around me married, had children, and bought homes, all I was doing was fighting cancer—stuck on a loop, the carousel. My life didn't look anything like I thought it would.

And so, I had to say goodbye.

Grief isn't linear: some days are up, and some days are down. I released my ideas of what I thought life would be. I released the resentment I had from how my life seemed to be unfair. I said goodbye to it all. Goodbye to my two-tittied life. Goodbye to life without multiple doctor's appointments. Goodbye to a life without medication. Goodbye to a life without pain. Goodbye.

Time to say hello.

Hello to the woman who, against all odds, stayed in Paris while facing a life-threatening disease. Hello to the woman who came to France without any French but now speaks medical French better than some of her French friends. Hello to a life where I take more risks and enjoy the small moments even more. Hello to taking special care to do things people may take for granted—like having a child or even breastfeeding that child. Hello to the woman whose story is not just surviving cancer, but everything that comes along with it. Hello to the woman who dealt with the ups and downs of expat life—mice, job searching, dating, miscommunications, apartment woes—and can now laugh about it.

I not only survived cancer, but I also survived Paris.

It would be so easy to hate France. Did France give me cancer? I didn't have these problems in America. "Why are you still living in France? Everything seems so hard there," friends asked me. It seemed to them almost like a form of Stockholm syndrome. It would be easy to make France—Paris, to be exact—the villain in my life story. But for all my woes, I would never do that.

My two battles with cancer bonded me to France more than I ever thought was possible. France is the country that took care of me at my lowest moments. America made me but France saved me. This was the place where people dried my tears and calmed my fears. It's the place that took care of me during the most transformative and defining experience in my life. It's the place where I learned what I was made of. It's the place where I eventually became a citizen, proudly singing *"La Marseillaise."* It's the place where I moved into a calm apartment with an Eiffel Tower view—after a long search to move out of the crematorium apartment, I finally found my oasis.

I moved to France because I wanted to create a different type of life—one where I worked internationally. I didn't expect this type of life. As I cried in my apartment in Harlem on the day of my move, this wasn't the fear I had for my life in Paris. My biggest fear was not finding a job or having to return home—but now I have two homes. If I knew this was in the cards for me, would I have still done it? Definitely. Before, I had lived a life defined by a set of rules and standards: things I put in place to make sure I was always prepared for the worst. And yet I wasn't prepared—not by a long shot.

It was hard to believe that my meeting with Rachel, sitting in her office essentially begging for answers, led to me living a life beyond my wildest dreams—and nightmares. Her advice was tough, but it was what I needed to push me beyond my comfort zone. I was afraid but still took the leap. I'm glad I didn't let fear hold me back. In the end, I found out you can move abroad, change your life, and do all the right things and the worst can still come for you. And Paris taught me I'm stronger than I ever believed.

• • •

LIFE IS SHORT BUT IT'S also long.

"30 under 30," "40 under 40": The lists show the "top" people in their industries who have all done it at such a young age! We should all aspire to be like these people—people who stayed on a path to reach renown only a few years out of college.

Or should we?

Society makes us believe if you're not doing everything by a certain age, it's a wrap for you. So meet those milestones—hit the ground running to start that company so you too can be on a "40 under 40" list.

This pervasive mindset hits particularly hard as a cancer survivor. I aspired to be on those lists, to have my name in lights. Except at thirty-four I was diagnosed with cancer, pausing my life for five years. Now, at thirty-nine, what hope do I have? I guess there's always "50 under 50" to shoot for.

It's true you should seize the day, take risks, and do what you want before our borrowed time is up. And life may be short, but my cancer journey made me realize life is long.

My life now is absolutely nothing like it was last year. And last year was nothing like 2016, years ago, when I was a newly arrived American in Paris. It's a massive change from where my life was years before, in NYC, traveling for work and enjoying Saturday brunches.

In a way, I feel I have lived multiple lives. Robin in Maryland wasn't the same woman as Robin in NYC or even the woman writing this in the 2nd arrondissement of Paris.

Life can change in an instant. Mine did. In a doctor's office, in a car accident, in a meeting with your boss, in the bathroom looking down at a positive pregnancy test. The elevator of life can be a wild ride of ups and downs. But change doesn't mean the end.

Looking back on my life changes throughout the years—violent, quick, massive changes—you never forget the changes themselves, but in time, the emotions around them are harder to recall. The fear, the pain, the sadness, none of it's forgotten, but it's easier to push past.

The anxiety about a recurrence still lingers—a feeling that I'm open about. My oncologist pulled me aside at my quarterly oncology appointment before leaving. "You have to choose hope every day. It won't be easy, it's a mental thing—but know that the treatment you did worked. And believe in that and choose hope every day—that you'll be as healthy in ten years as you are today."

That's not to say it's not still messy. After all the work I did, desperate to be seen as a good employee, a good worker, at my job—I was unceremoniously laid off. And the worst part? They called me while I was on vacation to tell me (yes, reader, I did indeed get "fired on my day off"—shout out to "Friday"). What was the point of it all? Of all the worry, the anxiety, the fear of taking too many sick days, the pain while sitting at my desk with a smile, the days I could barely face the world but still showed up ready to work? It meant everything to me—it meant nothing to them.

And sometimes, grief hits me like a brick. I saw the musical *Hamilton* in London with a friend. At the end of the show, the entire cast hits the stage for one last musical number, "Who Lives, Who Dies, Who Tells Your Story."

As the cast sang the refrain repeatedly, my chest tightened and sweat beads began appearing on the back of my neck. Who lives, who dies, who will tell *my* story?

Unbeknownst to my friend seated next to me, in my cushioned seat in London's West End, I had a full-on panic attack. This was a series of questions I'd asked myself so many times. A series of questions that kept me awake at night. If the cancer took me, a single and childless woman, who *would* tell my story? Would anyone even remember me?

In May 2021, twelve months after the beginning of my second cancer battle, nearly two years since I'd seen my family, I stepped off the plane at Dulles Airport in Virginia. I smiled. After everything I'd been through, it didn't feel real to be back on American soil. I pushed through the throng of masked faces, walking the long hallways to the People Mover and then to customs and immigration. The US border agent asked me from behind thick glass to lower my mask. I gave him a quick smile and he stamped my passport. "Welcome home," he said, sliding it across to me.

As I walked through the archway from customs toward the exit, I saw a familiar face walking the long hallway. My mother, wearing an N95 mask, jeans, and a button-up shirt spotted me. She picked up the pace, breaking into a shuffling run. "Mom, stop running, stop running," I yelled, worried about my seventy-something-year-old mother slipping and falling on the linoleum airport floor.

Luggage trailing behind me, I ran toward her to shorten the gap and we embraced. My father joined us, hugging me tightly. My sister squeezed me outside the airport, hopping out of the driver's seat despite the "move along" instructions of the airport police.

I landed heavier, tired, and with much less hair than the last time they saw me. But I made it. *We* made it: the Swiss Family Robinson was back together again.

Who knows what the future holds. So what if I didn't meet a Frenchman in the *supermarché*, so what if I never got the perfect international job, so what if I didn't have little children calling me *maman*. But whatever happens next, you know where you can find me. Sitting in my apartment gazing at the Eiffel Tower in the country that saved me and the city I made my home.

Acknowledgments

This book was several years in the making. I started writing it in 2018 after my first bout with cancer and dropped it. I picked it up again amid my second bout. Throughout these seven years, from start to publication, I couldn't have made it without the help of so many.

To my editor, Abby, thank you for seeing me for me! You understood what I wanted to accomplish and helped me dig deeper to get there. Makayla, you've worked tirelessly and held my hand through this process. I'm sorry for all my anxious questions! I appreciate you. Big thanks to the whole wonderful team at Amistad.

To my agent, William Clark, thank you for advocating on my behalf and getting us to this point. My early readers, those who pored over my proposal and early manuscripts—Juliet, Kelly, Jazmine, Anne, and Marissa (and for the title!)—thank you too.

I started this journey without a writing community and gained such a large one. Lori Tharps, thank you for your guidance, words of affirmation, and community building.

I hope I'm making you proud! See you in The Sanctuary. To my Sister Scribes—Kirsten, Tamar, Rolanda, Lisette, Christina, Linda, Kathy, and Hadiya—you've all been a positive addition to my life and helped me grow as a writer. Y'all got next! To Joy, Jeanetta, and my Black Women Writers in Europe sisters, thank you for the community and encouragement.

Cindy, Lyneka, and Izzy—I don't know how I would have made it without y'all. You three were by my side in my worst moments, and I'm eternally grateful. I'm so lucky to have friends like you. Shirley—you're an angel. Thanks for being there.

To Joi and Lauren, thanks for being my biggest cheerleaders—not just for the book but for the past thirty years. To my NYC girls: you've been an incredible sounding board and helped when my memory failed me. Thanks to Traci, Cassandra, Whitney, and Reniqua, especially for your transparency on the publishing world.

So many others stepped up for me—whether by dropping by for a hallway chat, sending food, sitting with me after chemo, chipping in for supplies, inviting me for meals, or in many other ways. Thanks to Nancy, Alexis, Clara, Chris, Ruochen, Kristi, Liz, Catherine, Mary, CJ, Dickas, Shweta, Jummy, Jules, Alisha, Brice, Caitlin, Cara, Juliet, Holly, Nicola, and Sarissa. Thank you to my church families of From the Heart and Renaissance for the prayers sent.

Of course, I wouldn't be here to finish this book without my medical team. Thank you for everything. To A, you

ACKNOWLEDGMENTS

believed in me even when I didn't believe in myself. Thank you for supporting and encouraging me.

Finally, to the "Swiss Family Robinson." I'm so blessed to have been born into this family. To Crystal, my sister, my first friend, and first editor—I can't say thank you enough for all you've done for me. Your feedback on the book was priceless, and your love and support have held me up on days when I wanted to quit—both chemo and writing. *Thank you*. To my parents, thanks for the love, the prayers, the flights to and from Paris, the long FaceTimes, and so much more.

To anyone I forgot to shout out, charge it to the head, not the heart.

About the Author

ROBIN ALLISON DAVIS is an Emmy Award–winning journalist, writer, and producer based in Paris and born and raised in the Washington, DC, area. After a ten-year television career in New York City and desiring to see more of the world, she moved to Paris in 2016 to pursue the dream of a more international lifestyle. She is a two-time breast cancer survivor; *Surviving Paris* is her first book.